An Atlas of
ENDOMETRIOSIS
Third Edition

Edited by

Caroline Overton MBBS MD MRCOG

Consultant Gynaecologist, St Michael's Hospital and
University of Bristol, UK

Colin Davis MD MRCOG

Consultant Obstetrician and Gynaecologist, Specialist, St Bartholomew's Hospital
London, UK

Lindsay McMillan FRCOG

Consultant Gynaecologist, Portland Hospital
London, UK

Robert W Shaw CBE MD FRCOG

Immediate Past President of the World Endometriosis Society;
Head of Obstetrics and Gynaecology, University of Nottingham
Derby City General Hospital, and Head of School of Human Development,
University of Nottingham, UK

Foreword by
Charles Koh MD FACOG FRCOG

Reproductive Specialty Center,
Milwaukee, WI, USA

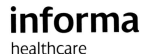

informa
healthcare

First published in United Kingdom in 1993 by The Parthenon Publishing Group.
Second edition published in 2002 by The Parthenon Publishing Group.

Third edition published in the United Kingdom in 2007 by Informa Healthcare, Telephone House, 69-77 Paul Street, London, EC2A 4LQ. Informa Healthcare is a trading division of Informa UK Ltd. Registered Office, 37/41 Mortimer Street, London W1T 3JH. Registered in England and Wales number 1072954.

Tel: +44 (0)20 7017 5000
Fax: +44 (0)20 7017 6336
Website: www.informahealthcare.com

A CIP record for this book is available from the British Library.
Library of Congress Cataloging-in-Publication Data

Data available on application

ISBN-10: 0 415 39573 9
ISBN-13: 978 0 415 39573 1

Distributed in North and South America by
Taylor & Francis
6000 Broken Sound Parkway, NW, (Suite 300)
Boca Raton, FL 33487, USA

Within Continental USA
Tel: 1 (800) 272 7737; Fax: 1 (800) 374 3401
Outside Continental USA
Tel: (561) 994 0555; Fax: (561) 361 6018
E-mail: orders@crcpress.com

Distributed in the rest of the world by
Thomson Publishing Services
Cheriton House
North Way
Andover, Hampshire SP10 5BE, UK
Tel: +44 (0)1264 332424
E-mail: tps.tandfsalesorder@thomson.com

Composition by Exeter Premedia Services Private Ltd., Chennai, India

Printed and bound in India by Replika Press Pvt Ltd

Contents

Foreword   vii

Preface   ix

Acknowledgements   xi

1   Aetiology   1

2   Basic science of endometriosis   5

3   Clinical features of endometriosis   9

4   Clinical findings   25

5   Classification and histological diagnosis   35

6   Ovarian endometriosis   45

7   Principles of treatment   51

8   Medical treatment of endometriosis   57

9   Surgical treatment of endometriosis   63

10 Ultrasound assessment of endometriosis   85
    Bill Smith

11 Nutrition and endometriosis   105
    Marilyn Glenville

Appendix   111

Index   113

Foreword

Endometriosis remains an enigma despite the many years elapsing since its description by Samson. It continues to defy research aimed at uncovering its etiology and the corresponding rational management that would result. Equally perplexing is the fact that afflicted women do not suffer the same symptoms and in fact some are completely asymptomatic. Research into the genomic characterisation of endometriosis may hold the greatest promise yet, and perhaps variable expression may explain the variable affects of the disease. But even this approach will see many false leads before the etiology is finally elucidated.

In the meantime however, the great number of women suffering from endometriosis need effective treatment now, and it is important for the gynecologist to be up to date in their understanding of treatment algorithms so that maximum benefit can accrue to patients, and just as importantly, that harm is not done from ignorance or employment of outmoded treatment.

The discerning student of endometriosis must fully understand the temporal evolution of knowledge when reviewing the literature and realize that much of the older data may not be extrapolated.

For example, the recognition of the various morphological appearances of endometriosis other than the classical 'powder burn', in particular the almost microscopic clear papule visible only by laparoscopic magnification, postdated earlier studies by laparotomy and unmagnified laparoscopy that reported the histological presence of endometriosis in 'normal' peritoneum.

'Deep' endometriosis was first defined in the early nineties, prior to which it was considered only 'scar' tissue and therefore not necessary to treat. Hence studies on surgical treatment efficacy and recurrence before this period should not, for example, be used in contemporary meta-analyses.

Fortunately, an increasingly sophisticated understanding of deep endometriosis is now present in centers that treat rectovaginal endometriosis with complete excision of disease to clear margins. In addition to providing longer term relief, such dissection also teaches the extent of such disease. In 2005–2006 alone there were nine papers on laparoscopic bowel resection for deep rectovaginal endometriosis, almost as much as in the previous 10 years. A very welcome trend in such specialized centers is the emphasis on adequate removal of disease, rather than resorting to hysterectomy and castration, the latter in my opinion being an overzealous surgical extrapolation of Samson's theory. This approach is a tragedy for younger women.

Hence to clinically understand endometriosis one must astutely sift through literature and disqualify papers that though well designed, were conducted at a time when little was known of subtle and deep endometriosis. Only thus can cumulative knowledge be garnered, leading ultimately to precise clinical understanding of the disease and its treatment. How does one begin on this path? Exactly by reading this wonderfully crafted text – the *Atlas of Endometriosis*.

In this third edition the authors have significantly updated the content to reflect current understanding, management and controversies resident in the treatment of endometriosis. The chapters are clearly written and will provide a basis for the understanding of current practice in endometriosis treatment for the student, trainee and practitioner. For the basic science researcher, this atlas gives a much needed summary of clinical information that aids their understanding of the clinical disease, thus providing substantive underpinning to their research at increasingly molecular levels.

This is a very comprehensive and balanced publication with up to date coverage of the theoretical, basic science, clinical, diagnostic and imaging, medical, surgical, and nutritional aspects related to endometriosis. It is more substantive than being just an 'atlas', but certainly demonstrates the strengths of an excellent atlas by including a very comprehensive array of photographic examples of surgical findings, imaging, histopathology and assisted reproductive technology.

Fertility treatment is brought up to date with contemporary evidence based considerations of surgery versus assisted reproduction in the context of success rates related to disease severity.

Pain amelioration strategies similarly give weight to contemporary evidence of efficacy of excisional surgery by laparoscopy, adjunctive measures like presacral neurectomy and the clear abandonment of procedures like LUNA. A clear enunciation of medical treatment in augmenting the results of surgery is well discussed.

The section on rectovaginal endometriosis excellently describes a once misunderstood and avoided area of endometriosis surgery, which often resulted in prolonged poor quality of life because of inadequate treatment. The authors' attitude mirror the recent immense interest among the foremost practitioners of radical endometriosis surgery in laparoscopically excising the disease completely, including bowel resection, urinary resection and repair if necessary.

The historical reflex of hysterectomy and oophorectomy as surrogate treatment of deep endometriosis is correctly questioned in the light of excisional data, and offers women hope of symptom relief without sacrificing fertility.

The authors are to be congratulated for producing this excellent atlas which is definitely recommended reading for the intended audience.

I can think of no better volume for the gynecologist, general surgeon, urologist, internist, family doctor to obtain a 'fast forward' to currency of their knowledge of endometriosis from the last time they learnt it as medical students. This allows them to more productively share in the care of the patient as an effective 'team'. This volume is also recommended for the resident, medical student and nurse wishing to understand endometriosis.

I thank the authors for the honor and privilege of writing this foreword and commend them for performing an outstanding service in the education of their readers on endometriosis.

Charles Koh MD FACOG FRCOG
Reproductive Specialty Center
Milwaukee, WI, USA

Preface

Endometriosis is arguably the most frequent problem encountered in gynaecology. It affects women in their reproductive years and has been described as second only to uterine fibroids as the most common reason for surgery in premenopausal women. The true incidence is unknown, but the study that came closest to identifying the frequency of the disease in the general population estimates that 6% of all premenopausal women have endometriosis.

Endometriosis affects women in the reproductive years, is associated with pelvic pain and infertility and, although not life threatening, can seriously impair health. It has huge economic and social consequences. The economic cost can be calculated directly in terms of health care resources consumed, and indirectly in terms of lost work capacity. The cost of intangibles such as suffering and reduced quality of life is impossible to quantify. The estimated total annual cost to society for all women with pelvic pain was calculated in 1992 to be £158.4 million (direct) and £24 million (indirect).

The first *Atlas of Endometriosis* was published in 1993 and a second edition in 2002. A third edition is required to update the atlas. Imaging, particularly magnetic resonance and ultrasound imaging, have developed, and new images are included. Advances in camera technology have resulted in greater clarity of the laparoscopic images, and images are now placed throughout the text making the atlas easier to read.

There have been significant contributions to the medical literature about existing medical treatments. A section has been added on new and potential medical treatments, as well as complementary therapies. A section has also been added on the natural progression of the disease, fertility and pregnancy. This remains the definitive *Atlas of Endometriosis*, covering all aspects of the disease and every question asked by patients.

CO, CD, LM, RWS

Acknowledgements

The authors would like to acknowledge the following contributions;

Dr Heather Andrews, Consultant Radiologist at the Bristol Royal Infirmary, kindly supplied Figures 4.18(a,b).

Mr David Bromham[†], kindly supplied Figures 3.8 and 3.23–3.25.

Mr Alpesh Doshi, Chief Embryologist at the Assisted Conception Unit, University College Hospital, London, kindly supplied Figures 7.8–7.13.

Dr Marilyn Glenville (www.marilynglenville.com) kindly supplied Chapter 11.

Dr Joya Pawade, Consultant Histopathologist at the Bristol Royal Infirmary, kindly supplied Figures 5.11–5.18, 7.14 and 7.15.

Professor J Scott[†], kindly supplied Figure 3.24.

Dr Basil Shepstone, Consultant Radiologist at the John Radcliffe Hospital, Oxford, kindly supplied Figures 4.19–4.24.

Mr Bill Smith, of Clinical Diagnostic Ultrasound Services, London, kindly supplied Chapter 10.

Professor Chris Sutton, Professor of Gynaecological Surgery, University of Surrey, kindly suppled Figure 9.64.

Figures 2.1, 5.1 and 5.10 are reproduced by courtesy of *Fertility and Sterility* and The American Society for Reproductive Medicine.

CHAPTER 1

Aetiology

INTRODUCTION

Endometriosis is one of the most common problems encountered in gynaecology. It affects women in their reproductive years and has been described as second only to uterine fibroids as the most common reason for surgery in premenopausal women[1]. Its true incidence is unknown, but the study that came closest to identifying the frequency of the disease in the general population estimated that 6% of all premenopausal women have endometriosis[2].

Endometriosis affects women in the reproductive years, is associated with pelvic pain and infertility and, although not life threatening, can seriously impair health. It has huge economic and social consequences. The economic cost can be calculated directly in terms of health care resources consumed, and indirectly in terms of lost work capacity. The cost of intangibles such as suffering and reduced quality of life, is impossible to quantify. The estimated total annual cost to society for all women with pelvic pain was calculated to be £158.4 million (direct) and £24 million (indirect). The estimated total lifetime treatment costs for a 1-year incidence cohort of women with pelvic pain is £10.5 million (direct) and £2.6 million (indirect)[3].

Endometriosis affects 45–70% of adolescents with chronic pelvic pain[4]. In a large survey of over 70 000 adolescent women, dysmenorrhoea was a common cause of reported school absence[5]. In the United States, chronic pelvic pain affects approximately one in seven women, with very high associated annual health costs[6]. A Norwegian study demonstrated that 2% of women had been treated for this condition by the age of 40[7]. Endometriosis-associated pain may be found in up to 60% of women with dysmenorrhoea and 40–50% of women with pelvic pain and dyspareunia[8]. Despite the identification of symptoms there is often a delay in establishing a diagnosis of endometriosis and hence a delay in ensuring effective treatment. This delay is on average between 6 and 7 years, and a consistent feature of most female populations[9].

Endometriosis is characterised by the presence, outside the endometrial cavity, of tissue that is morphologically and biologically similar to normal endometrium. This ectopic endometrial tissue responds to ovarian hormones undergoing cyclical changes similar to those seen in eutopic endometrium. The cyclical bleeding from endometriotic deposits appears to contribute to the induction of an inflammatory reaction and fibrous adhesion formation, and in the case of deep ovarian implants, leads to the formation of endometriomas or chocolate cysts.

The symptoms of endometriosis are variable and may be unrelated to the extent of the disease. The most extensive endometriosis can be asymptomatic and be discovered accidentally. Conversely, small lesions may produce marked symptoms. Pelvic pain related to the menstrual cycle, dysmenorrhoea and infertility are the major complaints of women with endometriosis, while menstrual irregularities and dyspareunia are also commonly associated with the disease.

The clinical diagnosis of endometriosis is primarily made at the time of laparoscopy, although there is increasing support for empirical treatment with laparoscopy if symptoms persist. The classic appearance is of blue-black lesions, but many subtler appearances are now recognised.

The term endometriosis was first used by Sampson in the 1920s[10,11]. He and Meyer spent their medical careers arguing their theories of pathophysiology. More than 80 years have passed, but endometriosis remains a perplexing and poorly understood disease.

EPIDEMIOLOGY

Endometriosis is primarily a disease of the reproductive years, and is only rarely described in adolescents (when it is associated with obstructing genital tract abnormalities) and postmenopausal women (when it is associated with obesity and exogenous hormones). No differences in the incidence of the disease between races have been found except for Japanese women, who have been reported to have twice the incidence of Caucasian women[12].

The exact prevalence of endometriosis in the general female population is unknown. Diagnosis depends on the observation of implants, at the time of either laparoscopy

Table 1.1 Prevalence of endometriosis by presentation

Women undergoing tubal sterilisation[6]	2%
Women with affected first-degree relatives[7]	7%
Infertile women[8]	15–25%
Women with surgically removed ovaries[9]	17%
At diagnostic laparoscopy[10]	0–53%
At gynaecologic laparoscopy[10]	0.1–50%
Unexplained infertility[8]	70–80%

or laparotomy (Table 1.1), and until a simple screening test is developed, the true incidence will remain unknown. There has been only one population-based study, which showed a prevalence of 6.2% for the disease[2]. Most prevalence studies have reported women presenting with one of several symptoms justifying laparoscopy, e.g. pelvic pain, dysmenorrhoea and infertility.

Delayed childbearing, either by choice or due to infertility, has been implicated as a risk factor for the development of endometriosis. The risk of developing the disease corresponds with the cumulative menstruation (menstrual frequency and volume over time)[13]. Women with shorter menstrual cycles (fewer than 27 days) and longer duration of flow (more than 7 days) are twice as likely to develop endometriosis than those with longer cycles and shorter flow.

PATHOGENESIS

The precise aetiology of endometriosis still remains unknown. It has often been called the disease of theories, because of the many postulated theories to explain its pathogenesis. The major theories of causation of endometriosis are the metaplasia of coelomic epithelium[14] or the implantation of endometrial fragments which reach the pelvic cavity by retrograde menstruation[10].

Transformation of coelomic epithelium

Dr Robert Meyer postulated the theory of coelomic metaplasia in 1919[14]. He proposed that endometriosis develops from metaplasia of cells lining the pelvic peritoneum. This theory is based on embryological studies demonstrating that Müllerian ducts, germinal epithelium of the ovary and pelvic peritoneum are all derived from the epithelium of the coelomic wall. If this theory is correct, peritoneum must contain either undifferentiated cells capable of transformation into endometrial cells, or differentiated cells that maintain the capacity for further differentiation. The rare case reports of endometriosis in men are taken as evidence for the theory of coelomic metaplasia. However, if the theory is correct, metaplasia should occur wherever coelomic membranes are present. Although there is embryological evidence that the coelomic membranes cover the abdominal and thoracic cavities, endometriosis is rare outside the pelvis. Lastly, if coelomic metaplasia is similar to metaplasia

elsewhere, it should occur with increasing frequency with advancing age. The clinical pattern of endometriosis is distinctly different, with an abrupt halt in the disease at the cessation of menstruation.

Menstrual regurgitation and implantation

The most popular theory is that proposed by Sampson in 1921. He postulated that fragments of the uterine endometrium, transported through the fallopian tubes in a retrograde manner at the time of menstruation, implant in the peritoneal cavity, giving rise to endometriosis[10].

The following evidence exists to support the theory of retrograde menstruation being the prime mechanism for the development of endometriosis: viable endometrial cells have been demonstrated in menstrual effluent[15] and have been grown *in vitro*[16] and even within the peritoneal cavity (in monkeys) if the menstrual flow is diverted to permit intraperitoneal menstruation[17]. Endometrial cells obtained from the menstrual effluent have been demonstrated to be transplantable to abdominal wall fascia[18]. The tubal ostia are located near the uterosacral ligaments in the pouch of Douglas, which are one of the most common sites of endometrial cell implantation[19].

Several studies have confirmed a high incidence of retrograde menstruation (90–99%) and the presence of endometrial cells in peritoneal fluid in women of reproductive age, and yet, only 1–6% of these women have endometriosis[20,21]. This suggests that retrograde menstruation alone does not give rise to endometriosis, but that some other factor(s) must be involved in its development. Those factors could include some alteration in the uterine endometrium of women with endometriosis, an altered immune response to retrograde menstruation or, alternatively, a more favourable peritoneal environment that may stimulate the growth and implantation of ectopic endometrium in the peritoneal cavity.

Genetic and immunological factors

Several clinical studies indicate that there may be a genetic factor related to endometriosis. The disease is more prevalent in certain families; the risk of developing endometriosis is seven times higher and more likely to be severe in women with an affected first-degree relative[22,23]. Endometriosis is more common in monozygotic than in dizygotic twin sisters, but no association was found with particular human leukocyte antigen (HLA) tissue types[24].

Dmowski and colleagues[25] suggested that genetic and immunological factors may alter the susceptibility of a woman to allow her to develop endometriosis. They demonstrated a decreased cellular immunity to endometriotic tissue in women with endometriosis. No clinically significant immune system abnormalities have been observed in women with endometriosis, and there are no differences in individual subsets of circulating lymphocyte populations[26].

Vascular and lymphatic spread

Endometriosis may also arise as a result of lymphatic and vascular metastasis, and explains vascular and lymphatic embolisation to distant sites outside the peritoneum, for example, joints, skin, lungs and kidneys.

Iatrogenic dissemination

There are numerous reports of iatrogenic transplantation of endometrial cells by gynaecological surgical procedures. Endometriosis in abdominal wall scars occurs after Caesarean sections, myomectomies and hysterotomies. Exfoliated endometrial cells collected from menstrual effluent have been shown to be capable of development *in vitro* and *in vivo*[18]. Menstrual effluent was injected into the subcutaneous abdominal fat of women planning to undertake surgery. The site of injection was excised for histological examination 90–180 days later at planned laparotomy. One of the eight women was found to have viable endometrial glands and stroma at the site of implantation, and another had fibrosis and glandular structures[18]. In a later study of seven women, one developed endometriosis at the site of implantation. Four others showed fibrosis and haemosiderin-laden macrophages and occasional glands, suggesting that endometriosis was developing[27] (Figures 1.1 and 1.2).

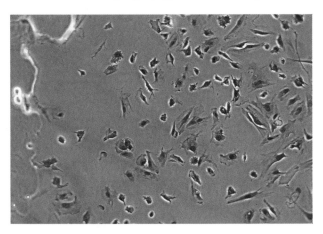

Figure 1.1 Stromal cells in culture

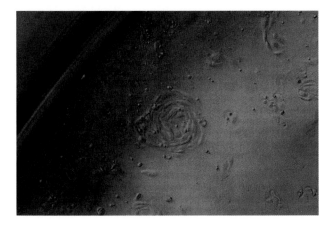

Figure 1.2 Endometrial glands in culture

CONCLUSION

On the basis of these data, the following hypothesis for the development and aetiology of endometriosis is postulated: retrograde menstruation, a phenomenon common to all menstruating women, transports shed endometrial fragments to ectopic locations. The cell-mediated, efferent arm of the immune system controls implantation or rejection of such fragments. In most women, endometrial fragments do not implant and are disposed of. In women with 'deficient cell-mediated immunity', implantation of the ectopic endometrial fragments gives rise to endometriosis. Such immune deficiency could be both qualitative and quantitative in nature, resulting in the variable age of onset, extent and kinetics of endometriosis, and could be transmitted genetically. Autoantibody production would be a secondary phenomenon in response to the ectopic endometrial growth.

REFERENCES

1. Detailed diagnoses and procedures for patients discharged from short stay hospitals in United States. Vital Health Stat 1984; 13: 86.

2. Houston DE, Noller KL, Melton LJ III, Selwyn BJ, Hardy RJ. Incidence of pelvic endometriosis in Rochester, Minnesota, 1970–1979. Am J Epidemiol 1987; 125: 959–69.

3. Davies L, Gangar KF, Drummond M, Saunders D, Beard RW. The economic burden of intractable gynecological pain. J Obstet Gynecol 1992; 12 (Suppl 2): s54–6.

4. Laufer MR, Goytein L, Bush M et al. Prevalence of endometriosis in adolescent girls with chronic pelvic pain not responding to conventional therapy. J Pediatr Adolesc Gynecol 1997; 10: 199–202.

5. Klein JR, Litt IF. Epidemiology of adolescent dysmenorrhoea. Pediatrics 1981; 68: 661–4.

6. Mithias SD, Kuppermann M, Liberman RF et al. Chronic pelvic pain: prevalence, health related quality of life, and economic correlates. Obstet Gynecol 1996; 87: 321–7.

7. Moen MH, Schei B. Epidemiology of endometriosis in a Norwegian county. Acta Obstet Gynecol Scand 1997; 76: 559–62.

8. Eskenazi B, Warner M, Bonsignore L et al. Validation study of non-surgical diagnosis of endometriosis. Fertil Steril 2001; 76: 929–35.

9. Husby GK, Haugen RS, Moen MH. Diagnostic delay in women with pain and endometriosis. Acta Obstet Gynecol Scand 2003; 82: 649–53.

10. Sampson JA. Perforating hemorrhagic (chocolate) cysts of the ovary, their importance and especially their relation to pelvic adenomas of endometrial type. Arch Surg 1921; 3: 245–323.

11. Sampson JA. Peritoneal endometriosis due to menstrual dissemination of endometrial tissue into the peritoneal cavity. Am J Obstet Gynecol 1927; 14: 422–69.

12. Miyazawa K. Incidence of endometriosis among Japanese women. Obstet Gynecol 1976; 48: 407–9.

13. Cramer DW, Wilson E, Stillman RJ. The relation of endometriosis to menstrual characteristics, smoking and exercise. JAMA 1986; 255: 1904–8.

14. Meyer R. Uber den Stand der Frage der Adenomyositis und Adenomyome im allgemeinen und insbesondere uber Adenomyositis seroepithelialis und Adenomyometritis sarcomatosa. Zentralbl Gynakol 1919; 36: 745–50. [in German]

15. Bartosik D, Jacobs SL, Kelly LJ. Endometrial tissue in peritoneal fluid. Fertil Steril 1986; 46: 796–800.

16. Mungyer G, Willemsen WNP, Rolland R et al. Cells of the mucous membranes of the female genital tract in culture: a comparative study with regard to the histogenesis of endometriosis. In Vitro Cell Dev Biol 1987; 23: 111–17.

17. Telinde RW, Scott RB. Experimental endometriosis. Am J Obstet Gynecol 1950; 60: 1147–73.

18. Ridley JH, Edwards KI. Experimental endometriosis in the human. Am J Obstet Gynecol 1958; 76: 783–90.

19. Jenkins S, Olive DL, Haney AF. Endometriosis: pathogenetic implications of the anatomic distribution. Obstet Gynecol 1986; 67: 335–8.

20. Halme J, Hammond MG, Hulka JF, Raj SG, Talbert LM. Retrograde menstruation in healthy women and in women with endometriosis. Obstet Gynecol 1984; 64: 151–4.

21. Liu DTY, Hitchcock A. Endometriosis: its association with retrograde menstruation, dysmenorrhoea and tubal pathology. Br J Obstet Gynaecol 1986; 93: 859–62.

22. Simpson JL, Elias S, Malinak LR, Buttram VC. Heritable aspects of endometriosis. I. Genetic studies. Am J Obstet Gynecol 1980; 137: 327–31.

23. Lamb K, Hoffman RG, Nichols TR. Family trait analysis: a case–control study of 43 women with endometriosis and their best friends. Am J Obstet Gynecol 1986; 154: 596–601.

24. Simpson JL, Malinak LR, Elias S, Carson SA, Redvary RA. HLA associations in endometriosis. Am J Obstet Gynecol 1984; 148: 395–7.

25. Dmowski WP, Steele RW, Baker GF. Deficient cellular immunity in endometriosis. Am J Obstet Gynecol 1981; 141: 377–83.

26. Gleicher N, El-Roely A, Confino E, Friberg J. Is endometriosis an autoimmune disease? Obstet Gynecol 1987; 70: 115–22.

27. Ridley JH. The validity of Sampson's theory of endometriosis. Am J Obstet Gynecol 1961; 82: 777–82.

Basic science of endometriosis

If retrograde menstruation is common, additional aetiological factors must be present which permit the development of endometriosis. These factors could include an alteration in the uterine endometrium of women with endometriosis, an altered immune response to retrograde menstruation or a more favourable peritoneal environment that allows the development of endometriosis.

HISTOLOGICAL EXAMINATION OF THE ENDOMETRIOTIC IMPLANT

Endometriosis is defined histologically as the presence of endometrial glands and stroma outside the uterine cavity. The use of the scanning microscope has altered the histological interpretation of endometriosis. Vasquez and colleagues described three different endometriotic implants[1]. The microscopic appearances are characterised on the basis of their relationship with the peritoneum and their endometrial glandular components.

Intraperitoneal endometriotic polyps with no gland openings characterise this first type, but these are associated with deeper endometriotic glands and stroma. The second, intraperitoneal endometriotic foci with surface epithelium, glands and stroma, presents stromal foci covered by non-ciliated glandular cells with gland openings. The third type cannot be detected by scanning electron microscopy because there are no surface endometriotic elements. The endometriotic lesions show only one or two retroperitoneal glandular structures surrounded by scanty stroma.

Laparoscopy does not distinguish between these three types, because only the sequelae of endometriosis are visible at laparoscopy: haemorrhage, adhesions, accumulation of fluid and inflammatory reaction. This explains the presence of microscopic endometriosis in peritoneal mesothelium that appears normal when biopsied[2].

Cyclical histological changes occur in ectopic implants similar to uterine endometrium[3]. Functional changes in endometriotic glands do not proceed as clearly or uniformly as in the uterine endometrium[4]. Compared with uterine endometrium, more than half of the endometriotic deposits were in phase with the endometrium, whereas in the remainder a dating was impossible[4]. This suggests an inadequate response to the ovarian steroids mediated by differences in the receptor levels, and may explain the unpredictable response of endometriosis to hormonal therapy.

The endometriotic implant reacts differently during the menstrual cycle according to the presence or absence of surface epithelium. In the presence of surface epithelium, the implant compares with the superficial endometrium, where, at the end of the cycle, the secretory changes are associated with arteriolar changes, necrosis and bleeding at the time of menstruation. In the absence of surface epithelium, the implant compares with basal endometrium, where proliferation, some secretory changes and vasodilatation occur, but there is no necrosis of the arterioles at the time of menstruation. In the absence of stroma, the atrophic cystic gland is enclosed in connective tissue, resulting in scar formation.

STEROID RECEPTORS

Oestrogen, progesterone and androgen receptors are all quantifiable in endometriotic tissue. Oestrogen receptors are at a lower level and do not have the pronounced cyclical changes that occur in endometrium. Studies of progesterone receptors vary, depending on the binding techniques or immunoassays utilised, but indicate a high level of biologically inactive progesterone receptors in endometriotic tissue. This is additional evidence that the hormonal control of endometriotic tissue is different from that in uterine endometrium, and may explain why a hormonal approach to treatment may not induce comparable changes in all implants[5,6].

FUNCTIONAL ACTIVITY

Although endometriosis is a benign disease, the endometrial tissue, after attachment to the peritoneum, has the ability to grow and invade the surrounding tissues. Similar to neoplastic growth, local extracellular proteolysis may take place, and therefore the fibrinolytic system may be involved.

An altered expression of several components of the fibrinolytic system in the endometrium and the peritoneal fluid in women with the disease has been suggested as a key factor in the establishment of endometriotic lesions.

There is evidence of increased fibrinolytic activity in the eutopic endometrium of women with endometriosis, resulting in endometrial fragments with a high potential to degrade the extracellular matrix and facilitate implantation. The peritoneum possesses an inherent fibrinolytic activity that is responsible for the degradation of fibrin deposits initiated after an injury. This physiological function allows repair of the mesothelium, and therefore prevents the formation of adhesions. The peritoneal fluid of women with endometriosis and pelvic adhesions has been shown to have an increased fibrinolytic activity that may be implicated in reducing the formation of new adhesions. Endometriotic tissue has abnormal proteolytic capacity. Proteolytic status is determined by the imbalance between plasminogen activators and plasminogen activator inhibitors, which are expressed differently in different types of lesion and at different stages of disease.

PROGRAMMED CELL DEATH

The endometrial fragments in menstrual effluent are composed of necrotic and living cells, which do not survive in ectopic locations because of programmed cell death. Augmented cell survival has been shown in eutopic endometrium from women with endometriosis. Cell death by apoptosis is reduced and cell proliferation increased. These changes may facilitate invasion of the endometrium[7].

Drug-induced apoptosis in endometriotic cells was attenuated compared to endometrial cells, suggesting abnormal survival in ectopic sites[8].

THE IMMUNE SYSTEM

Changes have been observed in both humoral and cell-mediated immunity in women with endometriosis. However, since all the studies have been of women with established endometriosis, it cannot be excluded that the differences are a result of the disease and did not necessarily predate it.

Changes observed in humoral immunity include mainly the finding of anti-endometrial antibodies in serum and peritoneal fluid. Multiple autoantibodies are present and suggest polyclonal B cell activation, which has led some to believe that endometriosis may be an autoimmune disease[9]. Changes in humoral immunity could, however, be secondary to deficient cellular mechanisms.

THE PERITONEAL ENVIRONMENT

Endometriosis is associated with chronic inflammation. Macrophage numbers are increased and more active in peritoneal fluid from women with endometriosis. Peritoneal fluid of women with endometriosis has increased levels of cytokines and growth factors that are involved in inflammation, angiogenesis and tissue remodelling.

The monocyte/macrophage system in the peritoneal cavity is thought to be part of a 'disposal system', the first-line of cellular immune response to the presence of endometrial cells within the peritoneal cavity[10]. Endometriosis may develop when the 'disposal system' is overwhelmed by high volumes of retrograde menstruation, or when a defective 'disposal system' permits implantation and growth of the endometrial cells or fragments[11].

CYTOKINES AND GROWTH FACTORS

These are polypeptides of high biological activity that were originally described to be produced by macrophages and lymphocytes, but are now believed to be also produced by epithelial cells, fibroblasts and many other nucleated cell types. They have multiple effects, including the regulation of the differentiation, growth and function of haematopoietic and other cell types. Cytokines are produced as part of the inflammatory process and in response to infection, but it is now known that they also have a role in normal cell physiology.

Interleukin 1 (IL-1) is elevated in the peritoneal fluid of women with endometriosis and in culture. Macrophages from women with endometriosis produce more IL-1 than those of controls[12]. Increased levels of tumour necrosis factor (TNF) have also been found in the peritoneal fluid of women with endometriosis[13]. The concentration of peritoneal macrophages in women with endometriosis was not correlated with the presence or level of TNF in peritoneal fluid, which suggests that peritoneal fluid is not the only source of TNF[13].

Recent studies have shown that recombinant TNF can inhibit the development of endometriosis in the baboon[14].

ANGIOGENESIS

Angiogenesis represents the crucial step in the pathogenesis of endometriosis, because endometriotic lesions require neovascularisation to establish, proliferate and invade inside the peritoneal cavity. Endometrial growth in hamsters appears to depend on cross-talk between vascular endothelial growth factor (VEGF), fibroblast growth factor and platelet-derived growth factor. The inhibition of VEGF resulted in a slight reduction in microvessel density when compared to control animals. Combined inhibition of all three growth factors significantly suppressed angiogenesis of endometrial grafts[15].

MALIGNANT TRANSFORMATION OF ENDOMETRIOSIS

Population-based studies have reported an increased risk of ovarian cancer in women with endometriosis. The fundamental features of human neoplasms (monoclonal growth, genetic changes, mutations in tumour suppressor genes and replicative advantage) have been evaluated in endometriotic lesions, but results obtained are discordant.

PROTEOMICS

Proteomics allows the comprehensive analysis of complex fluid and tissue samples with good sensitivity and resolution, and has promise in delivering markers for endometriosis.

Endometriosis-specific genes have been identified in the pathogenesis of endometriosis. The dysregulation of 14 genes was found to be overtly associated with endometriosis. Some of these genes, known to participate in oestrogen activities and antiapoptosis, may play a role in the pathogenesis of and may represent potential diagnostic markers or therapeutic targets for endometriosis[16].

REFERENCES

1. Vasquez G, Cornillie F, Brosens IO. Peritoneal endometriosis: scanning electron microscopy and histology of minimal pelvic endometriotic implants. Fertil Steril 1984; 42: 696–703.

2. Murphy AA, Green WR, Bobbie D, de la Cruz ZC, Rock JA. Unsuspected endometriosis documented by scanning electron microscopy in visually normal peritoneum. Fertil Steril 1986; 46: 522–4.

3. Roddick JW, Conkey G, Jacobs EJ. The hormonal response of endometrium in endometriotic implants and its relationship to symptomatology. Am J Obstet Gynecol 1960; 79: 1173–7.

4. Schweppe KW, Wynn RM, Beller FK. Ultrastructural comparison of endometriotic implants and ectopic endometrium. Am J Obstet Gynecol 1984; 148: 1024–39.

5. Bergqvist A. Receptor mechanisms in endometriotic and endometrial tissue. In: Shaw RW, ed. Advances in Reproductive Endocrinology. Volume 1: Endometriosis. Carnforth, UK: Parthenon Publishing, 1989: 53.

6. Bergqvist A. Steroid receptors in endometriosis. In: Thomas E, Rock J, eds. Modern Approaches in Endometriosis. London: Kluwer Academic, 1991: 33–55.

7. Johnson MC, Torres M, Alves A et al. Augmented cell survival in eutopic endometrium from women with endometriosis: expression of c-myc, TGF-beta1 and bax genes. Reprod Biol Endocrinol 2005; 3: 45.

8. Izawa M, Harad T, Deura I et al. Drug-induced apoptosis was markedly attenuated in endometriotic stromal cells. Hum Reprod 2006; 21: 610–17.

9. Gleicher N, El-Roely A, Confino E, Friberg J. Is endometriosis an autoimmune disease? Obstet Gynecol 1987; 70: 15–22.

10. Dmowski WP. Etiology and histiogenesis of endometriosis. Ann NY Acad Sci 1991; 622: 236–41.

11. Olive DL, Montoya I, Riehl RM, Schenken RS. Macrophage-conditioned media enhance endometrial stromal cell proliferation in vitro. Trans Am Gynecol Obstet Soc 1991; 9: 15–20.

12. Fakih H, Baggett B, Holtz G et al. Interleukin-1: a possible role in the infertility associated with endometriosis. Fertil Steril 1987; 47: 213–17.

13. Eiserman J, Gast MJ, Pineda J, Odem RR, Collins JL. Tumor necrosis factor in peritoneal fluid of women undergoing laparoscopic surgery. Fertil Steril 1988; 50: 573–9.

14. D'Hooghe TM, Nugent NP, Cuneo S et al. Recombinant human TNFRSAF1 (r-hTBP1) inhibits the development of endometriosis in baboons: a prospective, randomised placebo- and drug-controlled study. Biol Reprod 2006; 74: 131–6.

15. Laschke MW, Elitzsch A, Vollmar B, Vajkoczy P, Menger MD. Combined inhibition of vascular endometrial growth factor (VEGF), fibroblast growth factor and platelet-derived growth factor, but not inhibition of VEGF alone, effectively suppresses angiogenesis and vessel maturation in endometriotic lesions. Hum Reprod 2006; 21: 262–8.

16. Hu WP, Tay SK, Zhao Y. Endometriosis-specific genes identified by real-time RT-PCR expression profiling of endometriosis versus autologous uterine endometrium. J Clin Endocrinol Metab 2006; 91: 228–38.

CHAPTER 3

Clinical features of endometriosis

THE NATURAL HISTORY OF ENDOMETRIOSIS

The natural history of endometriosis is unknown, and well controlled experiments are difficult to perform because of the need for repeated surgical procedures to assess endometriotic lesions over time. Animal models provide an invaluable tool to study risk factors, prevalence and the natural history of endometriosis, especially in those menstruating non-human primates that develop the disease spontaneously.

The placebo group of women in placebo-controlled trials provides some evidence of the natural history of the disease. Endometriosis can both deteriorate and improve spontaneously.

A placebo-controlled trial of danazol and medroxyprogesterone acetate[1] (MPA) showed deterioration in 23% of those on placebo compared with none of the women on treatment. The disease improved in only 18% of women on placebo, compared with 60% of women on danazol and 63% of women on MPA. However, some of these women also had laparoscopic electrocoagulation initially, and therefore this is not a pure observation of the natural history of endometriosis.

Thomas and Cooke[2] reported a study of infertile women who had no other symptoms, i.e. no pain. Women were allocated to medical treatment (gestrinone) or placebo. Laparoscopy after 6 months showed that the endometriosis had improved or resolved in all the women treated with gestrinone. In the 17 women who were taking placebo, endometriosis improved in nine women, but worsened in eight, i.e. half improved and half became worse. In three women, this deterioration included the appearance of new adhesions around the tubes and around the ovaries.

In studies comparing gonadotropin releasing hormone agonist with placebo, the mean pain score was reduced significantly in favour of treatment, and most women discontinued therapy in the placebo group because of persistent pain[3,4]. The cumulative dysmenorrhoea rate was significantly less for the treatment group (7%) compared to the expectant management group (95%)[3].

It has been reported that 20% of women with unexplained infertility were found to have endometriosis 2 years after a normal laparoscopy examination[5]. This suggests that endometriosis is constantly appearing and disappearing in the pelvis. Evers[6] suggested that the impact of medical therapy in endometriosis is only temporary. He divided women who had equivalent amounts of endometriosis at the initial laparoscopy into two groups: the first group had a repeat laparoscopy in the final week of treatment and the second had the procedure delayed until the follicular phase of the second menstrual cycle after treatment was stopped. Resolution of the disease was significantly less in the second group, suggesting that the disease is suppressed rather than removed, and reappears when oestrogen stimulation returns. The evidence makes it difficult to justify the medical treatment of asymptomatic endometriosis when the disease appears ubiquitous and is not removed by treatment, and when it does not improve fertility.

CLINICAL SYMPTOMS

The symptoms of endometriosis are variable and often unrelated to the extent of the disease. The most frequent complaints among women with endometriosis are dysmenorrhoea, dyspareunia and pelvic pain. The pain is often cycle-related and increases premenstrually. However, it is not conclusive that endometriosis causes pain, as the severity of the symptoms has rarely correlated with the extent of the disease, and endometriosis is often found coincidentally during surgery or investigation for other gynaecological conditions, such as infertility.

The symptoms of endometriosis are similar to those of other common gynaecological conditions or disorders of the gastrointestinal and urogenital systems. Because of this overlap, many women with endometriosis have a delayed diagnosis of their condition and are often treated for other disorders prior to the definitive diagnosis. Women's self-help groups emphasise how frequently medical practitioners delay making the diagnosis, often because they fail to consider it as a diagnostic possibility. In the USA, it is estimated that 27% of women with endometriosis have been symptomatic for at least 6 years before diagnosis[7].

The diagnosis of endometriosis should be considered in all women of reproductive age who have cyclical pelvic pain that is worse in the premenstrual and menstrual phases of the cycle. Vaginal examination may reveal tender nodules of the uterosacral ligaments felt through the posterior vaginal fornix. The association of symptoms and tenderness on examination are often pathognomonic of endometriosis (Table 3.1).

ENDOMETRIOSIS AND PAIN

Frequency of symptoms

Table 3.2 summarises the frequency of the more common symptoms of endometriosis, compiled primarily from our own clinical experience but also from published data in the literature.

The annual incidence of pelvic pain in the UK is estimated at 14 000, with a prevalence of 345 000[12]. The exact

contribution made by endometriosis is impossible to calculate, because not every woman with pelvic pain will have a laparoscopic examination, but is estimated as 20–30%. The economic burden of the condition can be calculated directly in terms of the cost of health-care resources consumed and indirectly in terms of lost work capacity. The cost of intangibles, such as suffering and reduced quality of life, is impossible to quantify. The estimated total annual cost to society for all women with pelvic pain is £158.4 million (direct) and £24 million (indirect). The estimated total lifetime treatment costs for a 1-year incidence cohort of women with pelvic pain is £10.5 million (direct) and £2.6 million (indirect)[12].

Aetiology of pain associated with endometriosis

The aetiology of pain in endometriosis is uncertain. Given the poor correlation between most pain symptoms and endometriosis, only two conclusions are possible. Either endometriosis does not cause pelvic pain and a finding of endometriosis at laparoscopy is coincidental, or it exists in different forms, only some of which result in pain. Pain may arise due to the pressure it causes within the surrounding tissues, a function of its menstrual activity and location[8]. Thus, deep menstruating implants are painful if they occur within unyielding scar tissue and superficial peritoneal implants are not, as they usually expand into the peritoneal cavity. There is a strong correlation between pelvic pain and total volume of endometriosis ($p = 0.01$) and depth of infiltration ($p < 0.0001$)[9]. Pain may result from the local production of prostaglandins by endometriotic implants[10] or tissue damage and adhesion formation. Deep dyspareunia may result from pressure on diseased ovaries, uterosacral ligaments or rectovaginal septum[11,13].

Dysmenorrhoea has long been associated with endometriosis, and has been proposed to be a consequence of the disease. It was proposed that dysmenorrhoea was caused by prostaglandin-induced elevations in uterine pressure, and that the uterine pressure may increase sufficiently to alter the volume of retrograde menstruation[14]. This is particularly true if relative uterine outflow obstruction is present, and nulliparous women may be considered to have some degree of outflow obstruction in the absence of a vaginal delivery. According to this concept, dysmenorrhoea may be a clinical characteristic associated with higher pressures and increased tubal regurgitation rather than a consequence of the disease. However, in a study of fertile women, the incidence of dysmenorrhoea was similar in women with and without endometriosis[37], and cervical dilatation has never been shown to be therapeutic.

It has been postulated that the retrograde spillage of menstrual debris causes dysmenorrhoea, but this seems unlikely as retrograde menstruation occurs in 90% of women[15]. Prostaglandin levels in peritoneal fluid, menstrual

Table 3.1 Symptoms of endometriosis in relationship to site of endometriotic implants

Site	Symptoms
Female reproductive tract	Dysmenorrhoea
	Lower abdominal and pelvic pain
	Dyspareunia
	Infertility
	Menstrual irregularity
	Acute pelvic pain due to
	rupture/torsion endometrioma
	Low back pain
Gastrointestinal tract	Cyclical tenesmus/rectal bleeding
	Diarrhoea
	Colonic obstruction
Urinary tract	Cyclical haematuria/pain
	Ureteral obstruction
Surgical scars, umbilicus	Cyclical pain and bleeding
Lung	Cyclical haemoptysis

Table 3.2 Frequency of more common symptoms of endometriosis, as composed from analysis of 500 of authors' own patients and published data[8–11]

Symptom	Likely frequency (%)
Dysmenorrhoea	60–80
Pelvic pain	30–50
Infertility	30–40
Dyspareunia	25–40
Menstrual irregularities	10–20
Cyclical dysuria/haematuria	1–2
Dyschezia (cyclic)	1–2
Rectal bleeding (cyclis)	< 1

fluid, endometrium and endometriotic tissue have been measured in studies, with conflicting results.

Pickles and Clitheroe[16] first suggested that prostaglandins were involved in the aetiology of dysmenorrhoea. The mechanism by which prostaglandins cause dysmenorrhoea is thought to be direct stimulation of myometrial contractions[17]. Increased concentrations of prostaglandins have been demonstrated in the endometrium, endometrial washings and menstrual effluent of women with dysmenorrhea[18–21], and increased plasma levels of prostaglandin metabolites have been reported[22]. Prostaglandin synthetase inhibitors relieve dysmenorrhoea, correlated with a decrease in uterine contractility and menstrual fluid prostaglandin concentrations[23–26], and have been shown to significantly relieve dysmenorrhoea in women with endometriosis, compared with placebo[27].

Studies of peritoneal fluid prostaglandins are limited by the ubiquitous nature of prostaglandins and their short half-lives of seconds or minutes. Minimal trauma can elicit a large and rapid prostaglandin response, and studies measuring gross changes in prostaglandin metabolites may be inadequately sensitive to explain subtle differences in women with endometriosis. Luteal phase prostaglandin levels in peritoneal fluid were similar in women with endometriosis and controls[28,29]. Vernon and colleagues[30] proposed that prostaglandin production may be altered by the histology of the endometrial implants. Active petechial implants produce much higher levels of prostaglandin F in vitro than do inactive implants, although the prostaglandin F content is comparable. These findings suggest that in vitro incubation techniques may be a more useful indication of prostaglandin alterations than direct measurement.

There is no universally accepted hypothesis that explains how endometriosis can cause pain, especially in the case of minimal–mild endometriosis. Many investigators have proposed that women with endometriosis have an altered pelvic environment that interferes with fertility and provides the mechanism for pain. Data continue to accumulate supporting the role of macrophages in endometriosis. Macrophages present in higher numbers, concentrations or activation states may cause infertility by gamete phagocytosis. Activated macrophages may release factors that interfere with reproduction and activate nociceptors. Higher levels of cytokines, tumour necrosis factor (TNF)[31], interleukin 1 (IL-1)[32] and platelet-derived growth factor (PDGF)[33] have been found in the peritoneal fluid of women with endometriosis compared with controls. Fibrosis itself may lead to ischaemic changes. Unfortunately, there is no evidence in the literature to support any of these claims.

ENDOMETRIOSIS AND INFERTILITY

The nature of the relationship between endometriosis and infertility remains unresolved. Infertility is present in 30–40% of women with endometriosis, but it may be that uninterrupted menstruation results in endometriosis rather than endometriosis causing infertility. Although there may be some debate about the role of filmy peritubal or periovarian adhesions in infertility, it is agreed that with increasing severity of endometriosis, adhesions become more common and the chance of natural conception decreases. Even with severe endometriosis, natural conception is still possible.

The main factor that influences fertility is a woman's age. Fertility starts to decline rapidly after the age of 38, when the rate at which follicles disappear from the ovaries accelerates. In addition, the rates of miscarriage and chromosomal abnormalities, such as Down's syndrome, increase as women age. This biological clock exists for women because all the oocytes are present within the ovaries at birth. They undergo maturation and ovulation, but no new eggs are produced. A man can father children into old age because spermatozoa are produced throughout his lifetime.

Endometriosis and conception

Anatomical distortion caused by endometriosis, particularly in moderate and severe disease, reduces the chance of natural conception. With minimal–mild endometriosis, conception rates are similar to normal. If 100 women without endometriosis all start trying for a baby, 84 will be pregnant at the end of 1 year (Figure 3.1). For 100 women with minimal–mild endometriosis, 75 will be pregnant at the end of 1 year (Figure 3.2). For 100 women with moderate endometriosis, 50 will be pregnant at the end of 1 year. For 100 women with severe endometriosis, 25 will be pregnant at the end of 1 year (Figure 3.3).

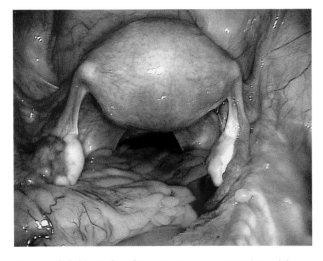

Figure 3.1 Normal pelvis: uterus in anteversion giving a panoramic view of the pelvis

Endometriosis-associated infertility

Adhesions are more common in moderate and severe endometriosis. They distort the pelvic anatomy, preventing oocyte capture. The pouch of Douglas is an important area in conception. If this pocket is obscured by adhesions, then the chance of pregnancy is also reduced. It is less clear why minimal or mild endometriosis causes infertility, where there are minimal or no adhesions (Figure 3.4).

If endometriosis is linked with infertility, then treatment of endometriosis should improve the chance of pregnancy. A large Canadian study found that surgical treatment of minimal to mild endometriosis increased the chance of natural conception compared to diagnostic laparoscopy. The method of treatment (laser, excision or diathermy) did not appear to matter[34]. The study was criticised because only blue-black lesions were recognised as endometriosis and

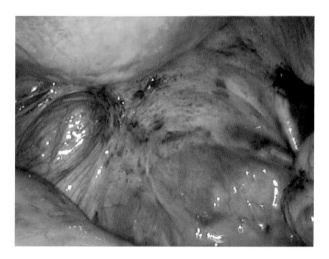

Figure 3.2 Active endometriosis on the uterosacral ligaments

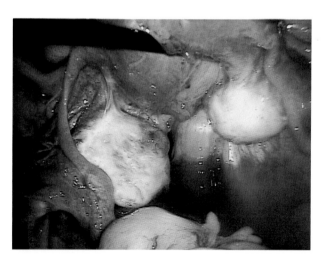

Figure 3.3 Severe endometriosis with both ovaries adherent to the ovarian fossae and the rectum pulled up obliterating the pouch of Douglas

subtle forms are increasingly recognised. The study also included women with adhesions, which introduced another variable.

Endocrine abnormalities (Table 3.3)

Luteinised unruptured follicle (LUF) syndrome is not an established cause of infertility in women with endometriosis. In this syndrome, the cycle is apparently normal, but there is no follicular rupture following the luteinising hormone (LH) surge. The unruptured follicle still behaves like a normal corpus luteum, producing a picture of ovulatory infertility. The association with endometriosis was initially made by observing the absence of ovulation stigma on the corpus luteum at laparoscopy in 23 of 29 women with endometriosis[35]. Further studies showed a higher incidence of LUF syndrome in moderate and severe disease compared with minimal–mild disease[36], and a higher incidence in women with endometriosis (75%) compared with fertile controls (21%)[37]. However, there is evidence that the diagnosis can frequently be made in fertile women[38] and in the luteal phase of conception cycles at laparoscopy[39].

Experimental evidence does not support reproductive endocrine abnormalities as the cause of infertility in endometriosis. These effects may occur secondarily to direct effects on the ovary, or the disease may secrete humoral

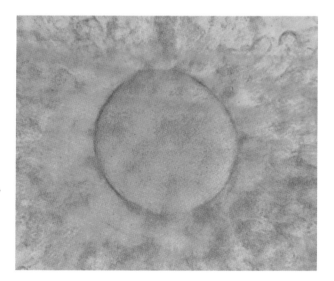

Figure 3.4 A normal egg as seen under a microscope

Table 3.3 Possible mechanisms of infertility causation with minimal–mild endometriosis

Endocrine abnormalities
Abnormal ovarian function
Adverse factors in the peritoneal fluid
Immune abnormalities
Abnormal oocytes
Spontaneous abortions

signs that directly affect the hypothalamopituitary axis. There is some evidence that LH receptor expression is abnormal in the follicles and corpora lutea of women with endometriosis[40]. There is also evidence that peritoneal macrophages from women with endometriosis may modulate the secretion of progesterone from granulosa and luteal cells[41]. The evidence in all aspects of reproductive endocrinology is conflicting, and it is unknown whether any of these defects results in decreased fertility *in vivo*.

Adverse factors in the peritoneal fluid (Table 3.3)

Fertilisation and embryo transport occur in the fallopian tube, which suggests that peritoneal fluid may not play a major part (Figure 3.5). Sperm survival is reduced in the peritoneal fluid of women with endometriosis. However, fertilisation occurs in the ampulla of the tube, by sperm that will not have entered the peritoneal cavity, and studies that show that peritoneal fluid is toxic to embryos can be criticised in the same way.

Immune abnormalities (Table 3.3)

None of the data are sufficient to suggest that abnormalities in humoral and cell-mediated immunity are causal in infertility. Anti-endometrial antibodies may impair implantation of the embryo. It is possible that the immune abnormalities may create an environment that is hostile to the fertilisation of the oocyte and the survival and development of an early pregnancy.

Abnormal oocytes (Table 3.3)

Fertilisation rates *in vitro* allow a partially quantitative evaluation of oocyte function and normality. Wardle and co-workers[42] compared the fertilisation rates per oocyte and per couple in women with endometriosis with those in women with unexplained infertility and tubal damage. They reported that the rate was significantly lower for both measures in the women with endometriosis ($p < 0.001$). They later reported improvement in the fertilisation rate following treatment of the disease[43]. They concluded that there may be an unknown functional defect of the oocyte that could mediate infertility associated with endometriosis. A meta-analysis of all published studies reporting outcome following *in vitro* fertilization (IVF) in women with endometriosis (1070 cycles) compared to women with tubal infertility (2619 cycles) showed that pregnancy rates per cycle were significantly lower in the endometriosis group (26% versus 36%, $p < 0.005$)[44]. Others show the difference only in women with severe disease, and explain this difference by the mechanical difficulties that result in the collection of fewer oocytes[45]. Analysis of the large Human Fertilisation and Embryology Authority database[46] indicates that there is no difference in outcome. The evidence supports the conclusion that the presence of endometriosis does not influence success on IVF or gamete intrafallopian tube transfer (GIFT) programmes unless there is mechanical damage (Figure 3.6).

Jansen compared fertility between women with minimal endometriosis and those with no disease on a donor insemination programme[47]. This is the only study that supports the observation that endometriosis affects fertility *in vivo*, with statistically better fecundability in normal women, and supports the proposal that endometriosis causes infertility. However, the study is limited because there is no detailed description of the indications for donor insemination. Conception rates after donor insemination are much higher in the partners of men with azoospermia than those with oligospermia. There were only seven women in the minimal endometriosis group, and the semen characteristics of the men may have been different from those in the

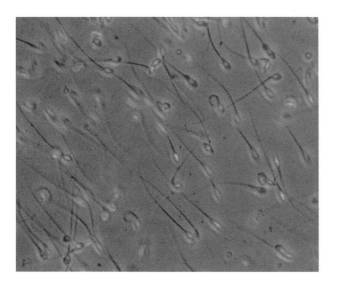

Figure 3.5 Motile spermatozoa

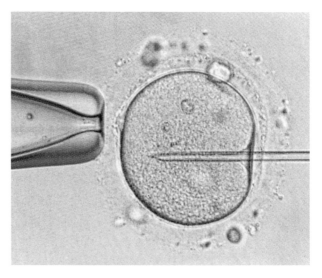

Figure 3.6 Intracytoplasmic sperm injection (ICSI)

control group, thus biasing the results. In conclusion, there is no definite evidence of an intrinsic abnormality in oocytes.

EXPERIMENTAL ENDOMETRIOSIS IN ANIMALS

Experimental endometriosis in animals has been shown to adversely affect fertility. Experimental endometriosis results in peritubal and periovarian adhesions that mechanically impede fertility[48], and abnormalities in the concentrations of peritoneal fluid prostaglandins in monkeys with experimental endometriosis have been reported[49]. Abnormalities of ovulation, including the LUF syndrome, have been described in both monkeys[50] and rabbits[51], while evidence has shown fewer ovulation points in rabbits with experimental ovarian endometriosis[52]. Autoimmune abnormalities have been described in monkeys[53], and an embryotoxic effect has been reported in rabbits, both in those with experimental disease and in normal animals injected with the peritoneal fluid from the experimental animals[54].

Although there is some conflict, good evidence exists that endometriosis affects fertility when experimentally induced in animals. However, care should be taken in extrapolating these animal studies to humans. Experimental endometriosis in animals is created by placing normal endometrium in extrauterine locations. There is increasing evidence in humans that the morphology of endometriosis differs greatly from endometrium, in oestrogen and progesterone receptor expression and in endocrine function. Therefore, endometriosis cannot be considered as just ectopic endometrium, and normal endometrium placed in ectopic locations cannot be considered to behave in the same manner as endometriosis. Spontaneous endometriosis has only been reported in the monkey and then at a low incidence. It has not been reported in any of the other animals, especially the rabbit or the mouse, which undermines the relevance of these models (Figure 3.7).

IMPACT OF ENDOMETRIOSIS TREATMENT ON FUTURE FERTILITY

There are many postulated mechanisms by which endometriosis may cause infertility. However, there is virtually no evidence to show that any are causal *in vivo*. This is due to the major methodological difficulties of demonstrating this experimentally.

Evidence that the treatment of endometriosis benefits fertility would provide evidence that endometriosis is linked with infertility. Medical treatment of endometriosis does not improve fertility. Thomas and Cooke have also shown that the elimination of endometriosis by medical treatment did not return fertility to normal[55]. The Canadian study reported a positive benefit between surgical treatment and future fertility, suggesting a causal relationship.

The relationship between infertility and endometriosis may be investigated further by analysing the success rates of IVF, GIFT and donor insemination programmes in women with endometriosis compared to those without the disease. The evidence suggests that the presence of

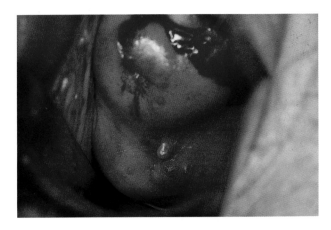

Figure 3.8 Endometriosis involving the posterior vaginal fornix. This deep endometriosis was continuous with lesions in the pouch of Douglas. (Courtesy of Mr D Bromham)

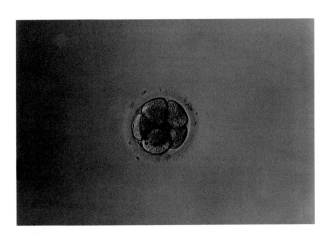

Figure 3.7 Normally dividing day-2 human embryo

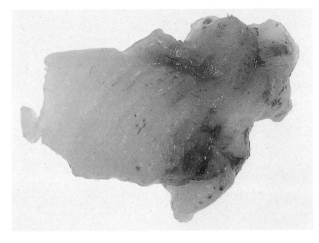

Figure 3.9 Excised vaginal vault endometriotic lesion

endometriosis does not influence success on IVF/GIFT programmes unless there is mechanical damage.

Pregnancy and endometriosis

There are case reports of exacerbations of pelvic pain during pregnancy. However, in general endometriosis has no associations with adverse pregnancy outcome.

Spontaneous miscarriage

There have been reports that women with endometriosis have a higher risk of miscarriage. These studies have been criticised, since they were retrospective and poorly controlled. In a randomised study of laparoscopic ablation of minimal–mild endometriosis, the miscarriage rate was 20% in both treated and untreated groups, which suggests that the presence of endometriosis does not affect miscarriage rates[34].

EXTRAPELVIC ENDOMETRIOSIS

Sampson[56] originally divided endometriosis into two main groups: direct or internal (adenomyosis) and indirect or external endometriosis. Current thinking is that internal endometriosis (adenomyosis) has a different etiological background. Additionally, external endometriosis is subdivided into pelvic and extrapelvic endometriosis. Pelvic endometriosis is defined as endometriotic implants involving the uterus, fallopian tubes, ovaries, peritoneum of the anterior and posterior cul-de-sac and pelvic side walls, whilst extrapelvic endometriosis is defined as endometriotic-like implants elsewhere in the body.

Extrapelvic endometriosis has been found in virtually every organ system and tissue in the human female body, and differs from pelvic endometriosis only in recurrence rate and anatomical location. Overall, the incidence of extrapelvic disease represents fewer than 12% of reported cases of endometriosis[57]. The frequency of occurrence decreases as the distance from the pelvis increases[58] (Figures 3.8–3.11).

Intestinal tract endometriosis

The intestinal tract represents the highest incidence of extrapelvic disease, most frequently involving the sigmoid colon and rectum, followed by the ileocaecal area and appendix. The small bowel and transverse colon are less commonly involved.

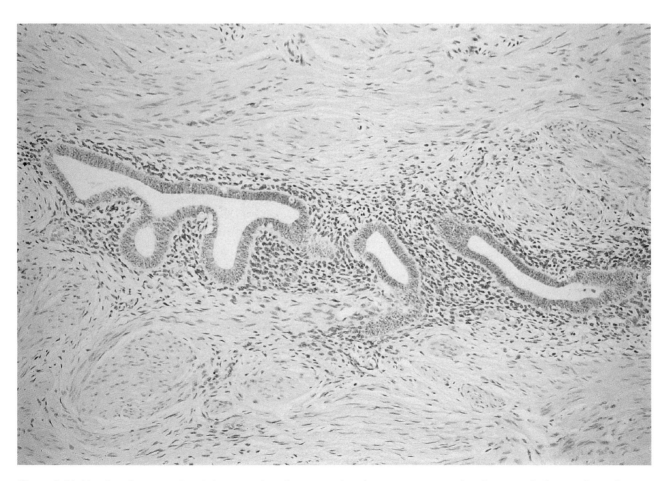

Figure 3.10 Histology from vaginal vault lesions, with endometriotic foci showing poor activity, but the patient had received gonadotropin releasing hormone analogues for 4 months preoperatively

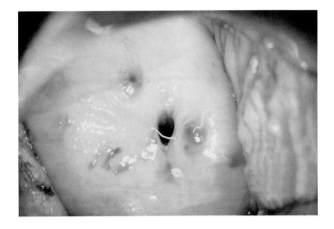

Figure 3.11 Endometriosis of the cervix

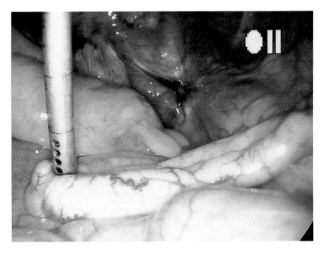

Figure 3.12 Hypervascular appendix infiltrated by endometriosis

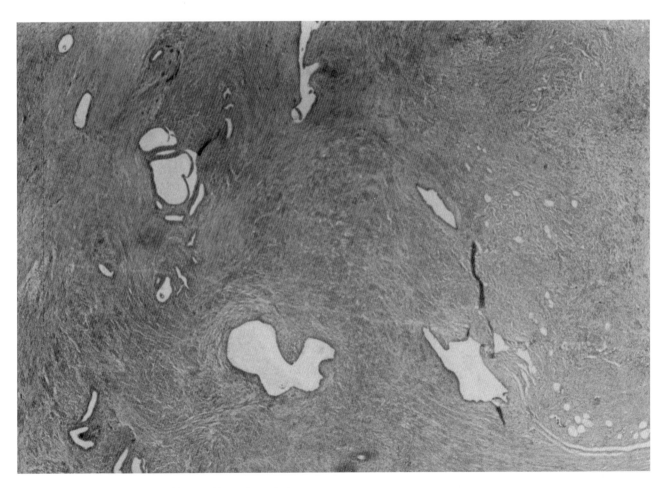

Figure 3.13 Appendiceal lumen obliterated by endometriosis

Endometriosis involving the intestinal tract without obstruction is most commonly managed with medical suppressive therapy. With increasing depth of invasion, the muscularis and even the mucosa become involved, and it is more likely that surgical treatment will be necessary, as the increased fibrotic response within the bowel wall often produces subacute or complete obstruction requiring segmental bowel resection.

Presenting complaints of women with intestinal tract endometriosis are most commonly abdominal pain, followed by distension, disturbed bowel function and cyclical rectal bleeding. Intestinal obstruction is more frequent in

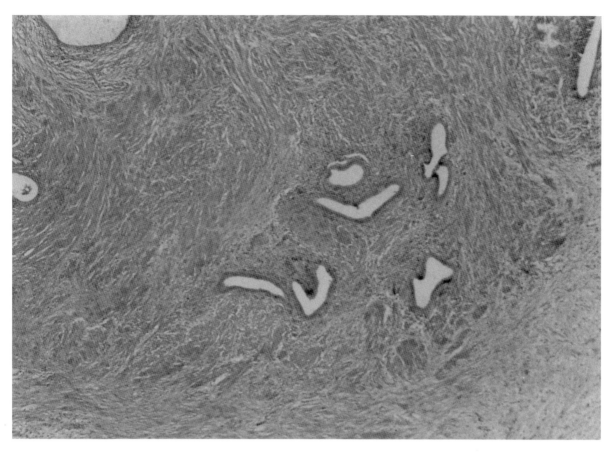

Figure 3.14 Appendiceal muscularis invaded by endometriosis

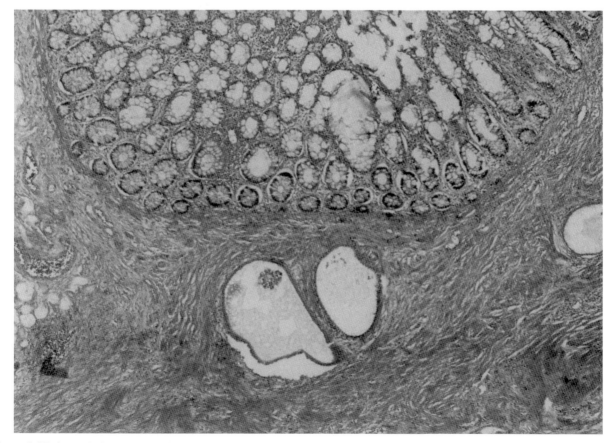

Figure 3.15 Appendical submucosa infiltrated with endometriosis

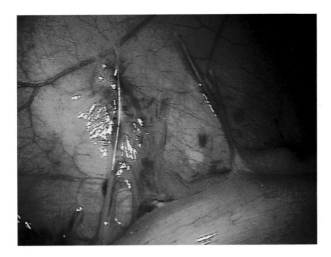

Figure 3.16 Vesicular implants on small bowel

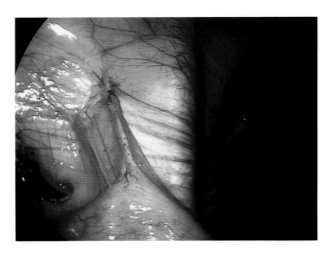

Figure 3.17 Small bowel adherent to the ovarian fossa

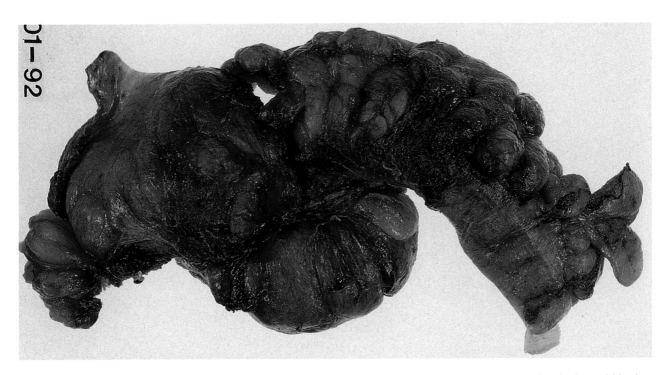

Figure 3.18 Endometriosis of the sigmoid colon. The patient (known to have endometriosis) presented with cylical rectal bleeding (perimenstrually), increasing dyschezia and tenesmus, and was admitted with obstruction of the large bowel

advanced disease and commonest in the rectosigmoid area (Figures 3.12–3.22).

Urinary tract endometriosis

Endometriotic implants of the pelvic ureter and bladder are less common than intestinal tract disease, but these are the next most common sites of extrapelvic endometriosis. Unilateral involvement of the ureter and kidney is the most common form of the disease, but bilateral involvement can occur. Endometriosis of the urinary tract may occur at any location, with the highest incidence involving the bladder, followed by the lower ureter, the upper ureter and lastly the kidney[59].

Common symptoms of vesical endometriosis are haematuria, dysuria, urgency and frequency, whilst renal endometriosis commonly presents with haematuria and abdominal pain. Ureteral endometriosis eventually induces partial or complete obstruction of the ureter and indicates the need for surgical management. The surgical approach wherever possible is segmental resection and reanastomosis or reimplantation of the ureter, although urinary diversion is sometimes necessary.

Involvement of surgical scars

The most common surgical scars involved are the umbilicus following laparoscopy, abdominal scars following

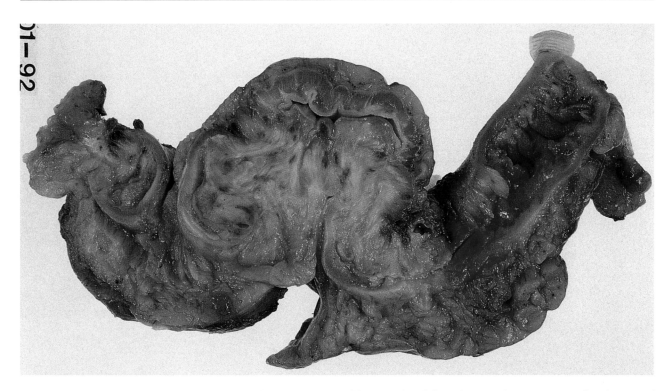

Figure 3.19 Stricture within the colon, increased fibrosis and polypoidal projection of the colon into the mesentery wall with areas of haemorrhage within the wall

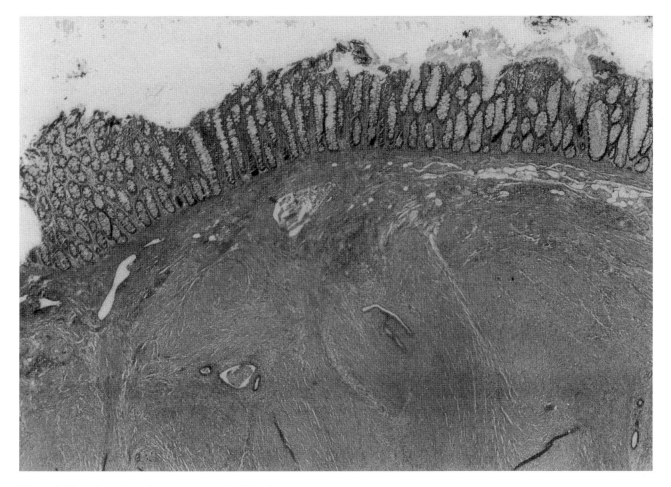

Figure 3.20 Colon with endometriosis invading the submucosa

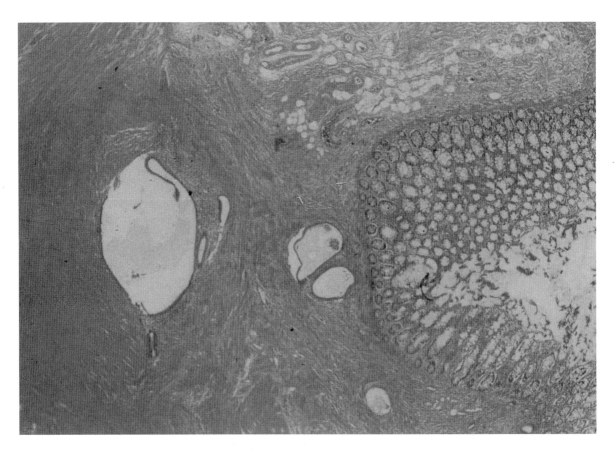

Figure 3.21 Endometriosis within a gland in the descending colon

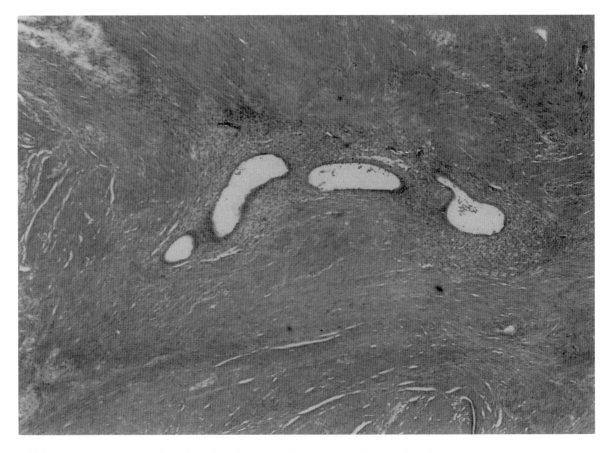

Figure 3.22 Endometriosis present throughout the colonic muscularis mucosa and surrounding glands

gynaecological surgery or Caesarean section and the perineum following episiotomy at childbirth. Most women present with a painful palpable lump, usually more symptomatic at the time of menstruation. Occasionally, women can be referred because of cyclical haemorrhage occurring perimenstrually. Medical treatment may control the symptoms over a period of time, but wide local excision is normally necessary (Figures 3.23–3.26).

Endometriosis of the vagina may occur following hysterectomy, usually when one or both ovaries are conserved, and usually in women with a history of endometriosis. It can also develop in women given unopposed oestrogen replacement when oophorectomy was also performed. With an intact uterus and functioning ovaries these implants are most commonly found in the posterior vaginal fornix. In most cases, these implants on the vaginal surface are continuous, with deep infiltrating disease in the cul-de-sac and rectovaginal septum. Whilst the visible implant in the vagina can be quite small, the full extent of the involvement can only be appreciated by bimanual pelvic assessment under anaesthesia, and it usually requires surgical resection either by laparotomy or laparoscopy.

Pulmonary and thoracic endometriosis

Endometriosis of the lungs and thorax represents an uncommon site of extrapelvic endometriosis. Diagnosis is usually difficult because symptoms of thoracic endometriosis are similar to those of more common pulmonary pathologies, and presenting symptoms and signs usually include chest pain, pneumothorax, haemothorax or haemoptysis, usually concomitant with menstruation (Figures 3.27–3.29).

Management of pulmonary endometriosis appears to favour surgical intervention with thoracotomy for excision of the implants and/or pleurodesis.

Suppressive hormonal therapy can be used as an interim measure and may help alter surgery, but with most

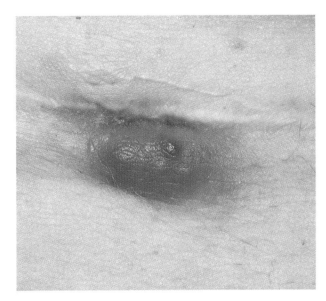

Figure 3.24 Superficial endometriotic deposit in Caesarean section scar. The patient presented with a cyclical, painful nodule on the scar. (Courtesy of Mr D Bromham and Professor J Scott)

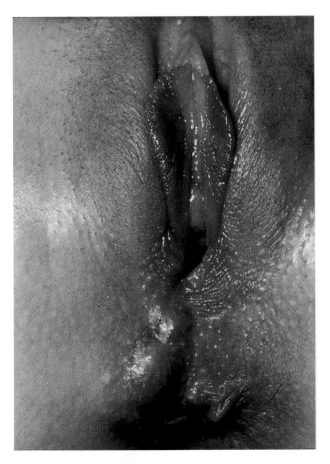

Figure 3.23 Endometriosis in an episiotomy scar. The patient presented with cyclical, tender swelling in the perineum. (Courtesy of Mr D Bromham)

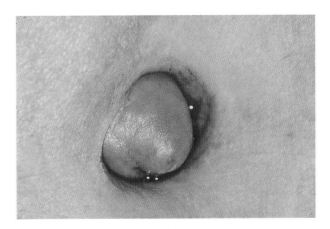

Figure 3.25 Endometriosis involving the umbilicus in a patient with extensive pelvic recurrent endometriosis. The patient presented with cyclical pain and bleeding from the umbilicus. (Courtesy of Mr D Bromham)

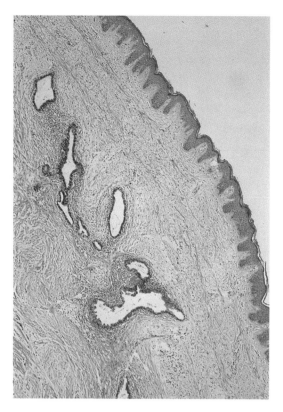

Figure 3.26 Histology of biopsy from endometriosis in the anterior abdominal wall showing glandular elements beneath the skin (H&E, ×90)

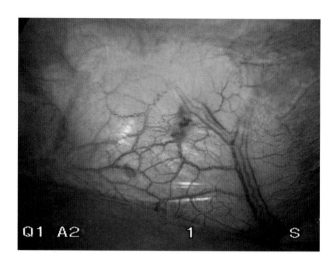

Figure 3.28 Endometriosis on the diaphragm with extensive neovascularisation

(a) (b)

(c) (d)

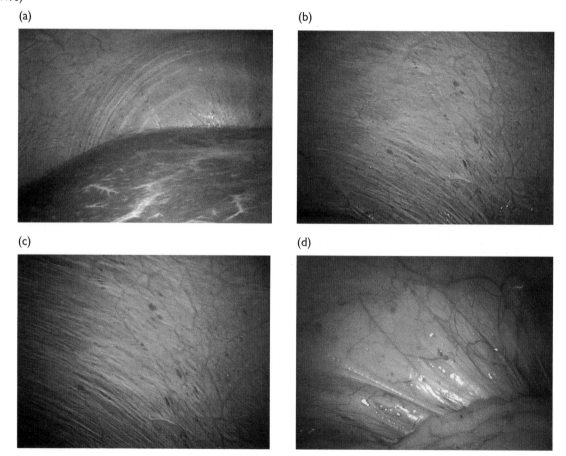

Figure 3.27 (a–d) Endometriosis involving the diaphragm

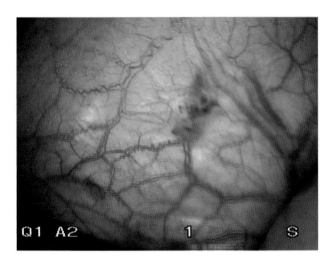

Figure 3.29 Higher magnification of Figure 3.28 showing diaphragmatic endometriosis with neovascularisation

deep-seated and extrapelvic endometriosis, recurrence following cessation of hormonal suppressive therapy is likely, making definitive surgery the preferred choice.

REFERENCES

1. Telimaa S, Puolakka J, Rönnberg L, Kauppila A. Placebo-controlled comparison of danazol and high-dose medroxyprogesterone acetate in the treatment of endometriosis. Gynecol Endocrinol 1987; 1: 13–23.

2. Thomas EJ, Cooke ID. Impact of gestrinone on the course of asymptomatic endometriosis. Br Med J 1987; 294: 272–4.

3. Dlugi AM, Miller JD, Knittle J. Lupron depot (leuprorelide acetate for depot suspension) in the treatment of endometriosis: a randomized placebo-controlled, double-blind study. Lupron study group. Fertil Steril 1990; 54: 419–27.

4. Bergqvist A, Thorbjörn B, Hogström L et al. Effects of triptorelin versus placebo on the symptoms of endometriosis. Fertil Steril 1998; 69: 702–8.

5. Pepperell RJ, McBain JC. Unexplained infertility: a review. Br J Obstet Gynaecol 1985; 92: 569–80.

6. Evers JLH. The second-look laparoscopy for evaluation of the result of medical treatment of endometriosis should not be performed during ovarian suppression. Fertil Steril 1987; 47: 502–4.

7. Kennedy SH. Report on the proceedings of the third World Congress on Endometriosis, Brussels. Lancet 1992; 339: 1532–3.

8. Sturgis SH, Call BJ. Endometriosis peritonei: relationship of pain to functional activity. Am J Obstet Gynecol 1954; 68: 1421–31.

9. Koninckx PR, Meuleman C, Demeyere S, Lesaffre E, Cornillie FJ. Suggestive evidence that pelvic endometriosis is a progressive disease, whereas deeply infiltrating endometriosis is associated with pelvic pain. Fertil Steril 1991; 55: 759–65.

10. Willman EA, Collins WP, Clayton SG. Studies in the involvement of prostaglandins in uterine symptomatology and pathology. Br J Obstet Gynaecol 1976; 83: 337–41.

11. Hayden GE, Söderstrom RM. Chronic pelvic pain: the diagnosis of endometriosis. Trans Pacif Coast Obstet Gynecol Soc 1977; 24: 128–31.

12. Davies L, Gangar KF, Drummond M, Saunders D, Beard RW. The economic burden of intractable gynecological pain. J Obstet Gynecol 1992; 12 (Suppl 2): s54–6.

13. Roddick JW, Conkey G, Jacobs EJ. The hormonal response of endometrium in endometriotic implants and its relationship to symptomatology. Am J Obstet Gynecol 1960; 79: 1173–7.

14. Schulman H, Duvivier R, Blattner P. The uterine contractility index: a research and diagnostic tool in dysmenorrhea. Am J Obstet Gynecol 1983; 145: 1049–58.

15. Liu DTY, Hitchcock A. Endometriosis: its association with retrograde menstruation, dysmenorrhoea and tubal pathology. Br J Obstet Gynaecol 1986; 93: 859–62.

16. Pickles VR, Clitheroe JH. Further studies of the menstrual stimulant. Lancet 1960; 2: 959–60.

17. Smith RP, Powell JR. Intrauterine pressure changes during dysmenorrhea therapy. Am J Obstet Gynecol 1982; 143: 286–92.

18. Willman EA, Collins WP, Clayton SG. Studies in the involvement of prostaglandins in uterine symptomatology and pathology. Br J Obstet Gynaecol 1976; 83: 337–41.

19. Chan WY, Hill JC. Determination of menstrual prostaglandin levels in non dysmenorrhoeic and dysmenorrheic subjects. Prostaglandins 1978; 15: 365–75.

20. Jones DE, Halbert DR, Demers LM, Fontana J. Prostaglandin levels in endometrial jet wash specimens in women with dysmenorrhea before and after indomethacin therapy. Prostaglandins 1975; 10: 1047–56.

21. Pickles VR, Hall WJ, Best FA, Smith GN. Prostaglandins in endometrium and menstrual fluid from normal and dysmenorrheic subjects. Br J Obstet Gynaecol 1965; 72: 185–92.

22. Lundstrom V, Green K. Endogenous levels of prostaglandin F_2 alpha and its main metabolites in plasma and endometrium of normal and dysmenorrheic women. Am J Obstet Gynecol 1978; 130: 640–6.

23. Anderson ABM, Haynes PJ, Fraser IS, Turnbull AC. Trial of prostaglandin synthetase-inhibitors in primary dysmenorrhoea. Lancet 1978; 1: 345–8.

24. Chan WY, Dawood MY, Fuchs F. Relief of dysmenorrhea with the prostaglandin synthetase inhibitor ibuprofen: effect on prostaglandin levels in menstrual fluid. Am J Obstet Gynecol 1979; 135: 102–8.

25. Csapo AI, Pulkkinen MO, Henzl MR. The effect of naproxen-sodium on the intrauterine pressure and menstrual pain of dysmenorrheic women. Prostaglandins 1977; 13: 193–9.

26. Henzl MR, Buttram V, Segre EJ, Bessler S. Treatment of dysmenorrhea with naproxen sodium: a report on two independent double-blind trials. Am J Obstet Gynecol 1977; 127: 818–23.

27. Kauppila A, Puolakka J, Ylikorkala O. Prostaglandin biosynthesis inhibitors and endometriosis. Prostaglandins 1979; 18: 655–61.

28. Rock JA, Dubin NH, Ghodgaonkar RB et al. Cul-de-sac fluid in women with endometriosis: fluid volume and prostanoid

concentration during the proliferative phase of the cycle – days 8 to 12. Fertil Steril 1982; 37: 747–50.

29. Rezai N, Ghodgaonkar RB, Zacur HA, Rock JA, Dubin NH. Cul-de-sac fluid in women with endometriosis: fluid volume, protein and prostanoid concentration during the periovulatory period – days 13 to 18. Fertil Steril 1987; 48: 29–32.

30. Vernon MW, Beard JS, Graves K, Wilson EA. Classification of endometriotic implants by morphologic appearance and capacity to synthesize prostaglandin. Fertil Steril 1986; 46: 801–6.

31. Eiserman J, Gast MJ, Pineda J, Odem RR, Collins JL. Tumour necrosis factor in peritoneal fluid of women undergoing laparoscopic surgery. Fertil Steril 1988; 50: 573–9.

32. Fakih H, Baggett B, Holtz G et al. Interleukin-1: a possible role in the infertility associated with endometriosis. Fertil Steril 1987; 47: 213–17.

33. Chegini N, Rossi MJ, Masterson BJ. Platelet-derived growth factor, epidermal growth factor and EGF and PDGF beta-receptors in human endometrial tissue: localization and in vitro action. Endocrinology 1992; 130: 2373–85.

34. Marcoux S, Maheux R, Berube S. Laparoscopic surgery in infertile women with minimal or mild endometriosis. Canadian Collaborative Group on Endometriosis. N Engl J Med 1997; 337: 217–22.

35. Brosens IA, Koninckx PR, Corvelyn PA. A study of plasma progesterone, oestradiol 17-beta, prolactin and luteinising hormone levels and of the luteal phase appearance of the ovaries in patients with endometriosis and infertility. Br J Obstet Gynaecol 1978; 85: 246–50.

36. Donnez J, Thomas K. Incidence of the luteinized unruptured follicle syndrome in fertile women and in women with endometriosis. Eur J Obstet Gynecol Reprod Biol 1982; 14: 187–90.

37. Lesorgen PR, Wu CH, Green PJ, Gocial B, Lerner LJ. Peritoneal fluid and serum steroids in infertile patients. Fertil Steril 1984; 42: 237–42.

38. Vanrell JA, Balsch J, Fuster JS, Fuster R. Ovulation stigma in fertile women. Fertil Steril 1982; 37: 712–13.

39. Portuondo JA, Pena J, Otaola C, Echanojauregui AD. Absence of ovulation stigma in the conception cycle. Int J Fertil 1981; 28: 52–4.

40. Ronnberg L, Kauppila A, Ralaniemi J. Luteinizing hormone receptor disorder in endometriosis. Fertil Steril 1984; 42: 64–8.

41. Halme J, Hammond MG, Syrop CH, Talbert LM. Peritoneal macrophages modulate human granulosa–luteal cell progesterone production. J Clin Endocrinol Metab 1985; 61: 912–16.

42. Wardle PG, McLaughlin EA, McDermott A et al. Endometriosis and ovulatory disorder: reduced fertilisation in vitro compared with tubal and unexplained infertility. Lancet 1985; 2: 236–9.

43. Wardle PG, Foster PA, Mitchell JD et al. Endometriosis and in vitro fertilisation: effect of prior therapy. Lancet 1986; 1: 276–7.

44. Lanadazábal A, Díaz I, Valbuena D et al. Endometriosis and in-vitro fertilization: a meta-analysis. Hum Reprod 1999; 14: S181–2.

45. Yovich JL, Matson PL, Richardson PA, Hilliard C. Hormonal profiles and embryo quality in women with severe endometriosis treated by in vitro fertilization and embryo transfer. Fertil Steril 1988; 50: 308–13.

46. Templeton A, Morris DJK, Parslow W. Factors that affect the outcome of in vitro fertilisation treatment. Lancet 1996; 348: 1402–6.

47. Jansen RPS. Minimal endometriosis and reduced fecundability: prospective evidence from an artifical insemination by donor program. Fertil Steril 1986; 46: 141–3.

48. Schenken RS, Asch RJ. Surgical induction of endometriosis in the rabbit: effects on fertility and concentrations of peritoneal prostaglandins. Fertil Steril 1980; 34: 581–7.

49. Schenken RS, Asch RJ, Williams RF, Hodgen GD. Etiology of infertility in monkeys with endometriosis: measurement of peritoneal fluid prostaglandins. Am J Obstet Gynecol 1984; 150: 349–53.

50. Schenken RS, Asch RJ, Williams RF, Hodgen GD. Etiology of infertility in monkeys with endometriosis. Luteinized unruptured follicles, luteal phase defects, pelvic adhesions and spontaneous abortions. Fertil Steril 1984; 41: 122–30.

51. Donnez J, Wayemberg M, Casanas-Roux F et al. Effect on ovulation of surgically induced endometriosis in rabbits. Gynecol Obstet Invest 1987; 24: 131–7.

52. Kaplan CR, Eddy CA, Olive DL, Schenken RS. Effect of ovarian endometriosis on ovulation in rabbits. Am J Obstet Gynecol 1989; 160: 40–4.

53. Dmowski WP, Steele RW, Baker GF. Deficient cellular immunity in endometriosis. Am J Obstet Gynecol 1981; 141: 377–83.

54. Hahn DW, Carraher RP, Foldesy RG, McGuire JL. Experimental evidence for failure to implant as a mechanism of infertility associated with endometriosis. Am J Obstet Gynecol 1986; 155: 1109–13.

55. Thomas EJ, Cooke ID. Successful treatment of asymptomatic endometriosis: does it benefit infertile women? Br Med J 1987; 294: 1117–19.

56. Sampson JA. The development of the implantation theory for the origin of peritoneal endometriosis. Am J Obstet Gynecol 1940; 40: 549–57.

57. Rock JA, Markham SM. Extrapelvic endometriosis. In: Wilson EA, ed. Endometriosis. New York: Alan R Liss, 1987: 185.

58. Williams TJ, Pratt JH. Endometriosis in 1,000 consecutive celiotomies: incidence and management. Am J Obstet Gynecol 1977; 129: 245–50.

59. Kerr SW. Endometriosis involving the urinary tract. Clin Obstet Gynecol 1966; 9: 331–57.

CHAPTER 4

Clinical findings

INTRODUCTION

The possibility of endometriosis should be considered in any woman presenting with infertility or with worsening dysmenorrhoea, pelvic pain or dyspareunia. There may be other cyclical symptoms, particularly related to the gastrointestinal or urogenital system.

The typical history is of pain which increases premenstrually, and severe dysmenorrhoea with the least pain in the follicular phase.

CLINICAL FINDINGS

Pelvic endometriosis

Clinical findings in endometriosis are markedly variable. In mild cases, routine gynaecological examination is likely to reveal no abnormality. A common feature of bimanual pelvic examination is that of discomfort, especially if performed during the premenstrual phase. It may be possible to palpate induration and tenderness in the uterosacral ligaments when these are involved (Figure 4.1). These features are demonstrated perhaps most clearly by a combined vaginal and rectal examination. If the pouch of Douglas is involved extensively, the uterus will become fixed in retroversion, and the adnexa will appear immobile.

Rarely, there may be bluish cystic lesions seen in the vagina and/or on the cervix.

Ovarian endometriosis

Deep involvement of the ovaries, with the formation of cystic endometriomas, may be suspected from unilateral adnexal tenderness, although palpation of a cyst of less than 5 cm in diameter may be difficult. The finding of a defined adnexal mass or unilateral adnexal pathology with tenderness in a woman of reproductive age is always suggestive of endometriosis (Figure 4.2).

Rectovaginal endometriosis

Deep disease is generally suspected when there are palpable nodules associated with focal tenderness on clinical examination. Examination with a speculum reveals either a normal vaginal mucosa or a protruded endometriotic nodule in the posterior fornix. By palpation the diameter of the lesion can be evaluated. Palpation is often very painful, and the presence of the nodule accounts for symptoms such as deep dyspareunia, dyschezia and dysmenorrhoea. The presence of the disease can be more readily confirmed by examination under anaesthesia for these palpable nodules. This is best performed by careful palpation of the posterior vaginal fornix, uterosacral ligaments and rectovaginal septum (Figure 4.3).

Bowel and extrapelvic endometriosis

When the mucosa of the rectum, sigmoid or bladder is involved, there may be overt haemorrhage, or haemorrhagic implants may be visible if viewed perimenstrually (Figure 4.4). However, in many instances, even with deep-seated involvement, there is no obvious mucosal implant. Bimanual examination may reveal areas of nodularity and fibrosis. Deeper implants of endometriosis may be felt as nodules using a blunt probe at the time of laparoscopy.

For specific diagnosis in the majority of instances, both visualisation and biopsy of the implants are essential, at laparoscopy and/or laparotomy.

SERUM MARKERS

Attempts have been made to use specific serum markers for endometriosis. The most widely used has been the measurement of CA 125, which is a cell surface antigen expressed in derivatives of coelomic epithelium, peritoneum and the endocervix. Measurement is by a mononuclear antibody to CA 125, which is raised against an ovarian epithelial tumour antigen OC 125. Women with endometriosis tend to have higher serum levels than do normal women[1]. Further studies have shown that, whilst a significant proportion of women with moderate and severe endometriosis have elevated levels, women with mild and minimal stages of the disease have levels within the normal range. Thus, the specificity when using serum CA 125 as a screening test for the presence of endometriosis is poor[2].

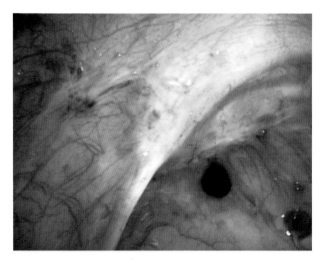

Figure 4.1 Black deposits on the uterosacral ligament with the uterus in anteversion

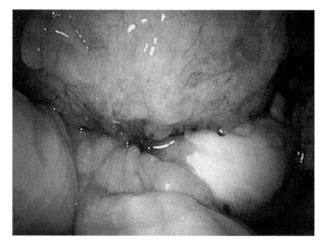

Figure 4.3 Rectovaginal endometriosis and obliterated pouch of Douglas

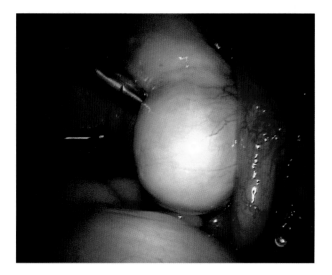

Figure 4.2 Right ovarian endometrioma

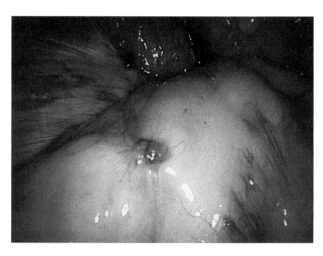

Figure 4.4 Endometriotic deposit on the sigmoid colon

CA 125 is not specific for endometriosis. It may be raised where there is 'irritation' of the peritoneal, pleural or pericardial peritoneum. It may be raised in appendicitis and pelvic inflammatory disease, ovarian cysts, pericarditis and pleural inflammation. Levels also increase in pregnancy.

Our own studies have found that, whilst measurement of serum CA 125 may not be helpful in the initial diagnosis of endometriosis, in women in whom it was found to be elevated, serial monitoring of levels was a pointer for the recurrence of the disease during follow-up[3].

CA 15-3 and CA 19-9 have also been explored, without much success.

Aromatase P450 messenger RNA expression

Aromatase P450, the enzyme that catalyses the conversion of C19 steroids to oestrone, is expressed in the eutopic endometrium of women with endometriosis. However, it is not specific for endometriosis and is also raised with adenomyosis, leiomyomas and endometrial carcinoma.

RADIOLOGICAL APPEARANCES OF ENDOMETRIOSIS

Ultrasound

Ultrasound is useful in the diagnosis and exclusion of an ovarian endometrioma[4] (Figures 4.5–4.16). High-resolution images may be obtained via the transvaginal approach using a 7.5-MHz probe. Sensitivity in the detection of focal endometrial implants is poor. However, the detection of endometriomas using ultrasound is excellent, with reports of 83% sensitivity and 98% specificity. There is a broad range of ultrasound appearances of endometriomas. Diffuse low-level internal echoes occur in 95% of endometriomas.

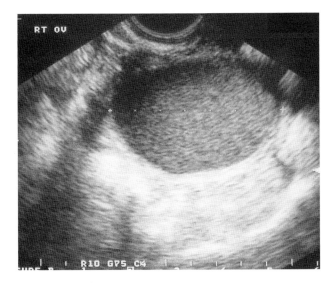

Figure 4.5 Transvaginal ultrasound scan showing the typical ground glass appearance of an endometrioma

Hyperechoic wall foci and multilocularity also point towards an endometrioma. Endometriomas are usually adherent to the pelvic side wall. This immobility is a useful diagnostic indicator.

In the case of deeply infiltrating endometriosis, particularly with deep deposits greater than 3 cm in diameter, there may be involvement of the ureter. Ultrasound provides a useful screening tool for hydroureter and hydronephrosis (Figure 4.17).

Computed tomography and magnetic resonance imaging

The pouch of Douglas is a potential space, and is not well seen by computed tomography (CT) unless distended by fluid or a mass. Endometriomas may appear solid, cystic or mixed solid and cystic, resulting in an overlap in appearance with an abscess, ovarian cyst or even a malignant lesion.

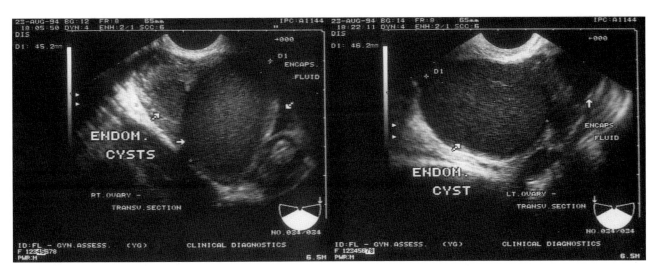

Figure 4.6 Localised transvaginal scans of both ovaries showing typical ultrasound features of bilateral endometriotic cysts. Pockets of loculated fluid and adhesions around both ovaries are clearly shown. Normal ovarian tissue is visualised within the right ovary

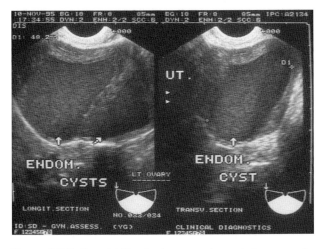

Figure 4.7 Differential bleeding into an endometriotic cyst results in a 'septate' appearance within lesions

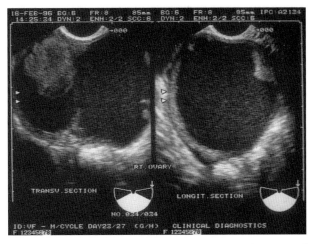

Figure 4.8 Differential bleeding into a previously aspirated endometriotic cyst can result in a 'complex' appearance

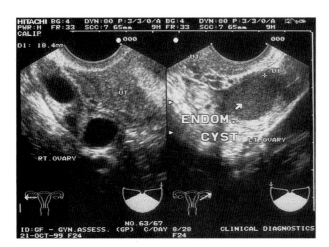

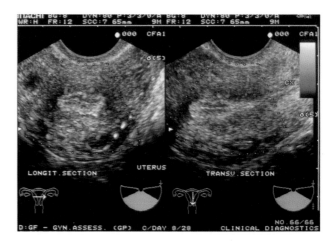

Figure 4.9 Transvaginal scanning shows an endometriotic cyst within the left ovary. The right ovary remains normal

Figure 4.10 Increased myometrial vascularity is clearly demonstrated by colour Doppler examination – this feature is often associated with pelvic endometriosis and remains very suggestive of adenomyosis

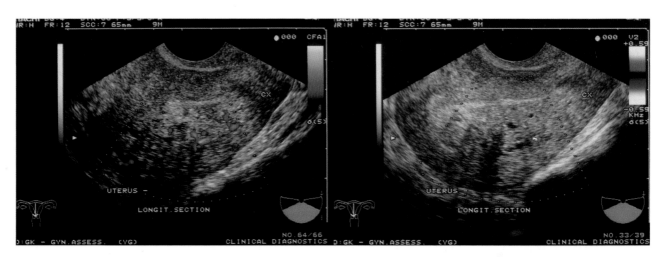

Figure 4.11 Parasagittal, transvaginal scans of the uterus reveal ultrasound features typically associated with adenomyosis. These include: differential thickening of the myometrium; irregular, mottled myometrial texture; prominent myometrial glands; poorly defined endometrial development with loss of the endometrial–myometrial interface; and increased myometrial vascularity

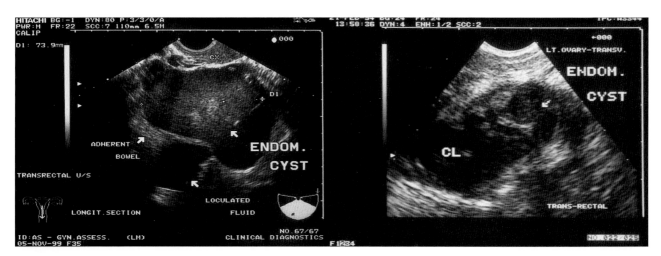

Figure 4.12 Transrectal scanning provides more effective imaging of the deep pelvis. Both images demonstrate ovaries adherent within the pouch region in patients experiencing severe pelvic pain and unable to tolerate transvaginal scanning

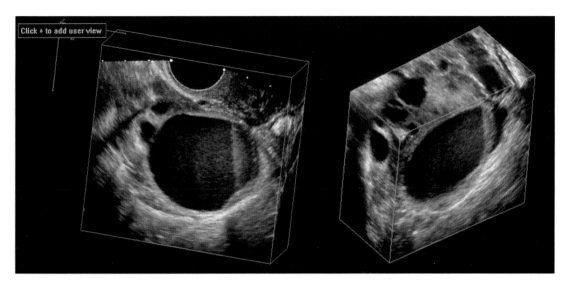

Figure 4.13 Three dimensional ultrasound: multisectional reconstruction and volumetric rotation of the ovary clearly delineate a single endometriotic lesion and its location within the ovary

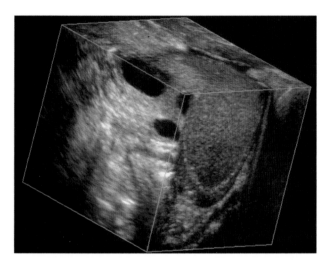

Figure 4.14 Three-dimensional ultrasound demonstrating a volume block of the ovary. An endometriotic cyst is clearly outlined within the ovarian substance. Normal ovarian tissue containing multiple antral follicles is very evident

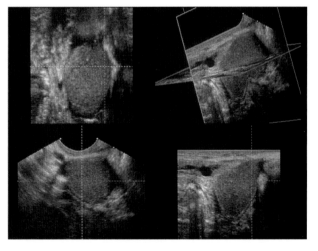

Figure 4.15 Three-dimensional ultrasound showing multisectional reconstruction of a large endometriotic cyst – alterations in the image planes confirm a lack of preserved, normal ovarian tissue

Owing to the poor specificity and high radiation dose, CT has been replaced by magnetic resonance imaging (MRI) in the evaluation of pelvic endometriosis.

MRI offers a look at the pouch of Douglas similar to that with CT, but with the added benefit of imaging in multiple planes. The pouch of Douglas region is especially well defined on sagittal images. MRI is a useful non-invasive tool in the diagnosis of deep endometriosis (Figure 4.18). It has limitations in the visualisation of small endometriotic implants and adhesions, but has the ability to characterise the lesions and to study extraperitoneal locations and the contents of pelvic masses[5]. The identification of endometriomas by MRI relies on the detection of pigmented lesions. Signal characteristics vary according to the age of

the haemorrhage. Typically lesions appear hyperintense on T1-weighted spin-echo (SE) images and hypointense (shading) on T2-weighted turbo spin-echo (TSE) images due to the presence of deoxyhaemoglobin and methaemoglobin. Acute haemorrhage occasionally appears hypointense on T1-weighted SE images and T2-weighted TSE images. Old haemorrhage occasionally appears hyperintense on T1-weighted SE images and T2-weighted TSE images.

Barium enema

The barium enema, particularly the double-contrast enema, offers an excellent view of abnormalities in the pouch of Douglas. The best views are the lateral or prone cross-table view of the rectum. It is possible to differentiate between

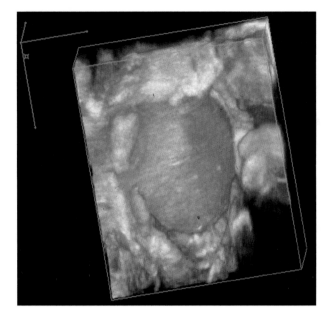

Figure 4.16 Three-dimensional ultrasound: surface rendering technique isolates 'in full 3D' an endometrioma contained within the ovary. A thick band of adhesions is partly visualised attaching the ovary and endometriotic lesion to the pelvic side wall. Adherent ovarian capsule is evident between the lesion and the pelvic side wall

cases in which the bowel is simply displaced by a pelvic endometrioma and cases with bowel involvement. Cases without bowel involvement present as smooth extrinsic masses, while those involving the bowel demonstrate a crenulated or tethered mucosal pattern. Endometriosis involving the bowel wall with crenulation is indistinguishable from a malignant tumour invading the bowel.

Sigmoidoscopy

Sigmoidoscopy is mentioned by the authors to comment that it is not a useful preoperative test for rectovaginal endometriosis. Rectovaginal endometriosis is suspected by the clinical history of dyschezia and clinical examination.

OC 125 immunoscintigraphy

Immunoscintigraphy with ^{131}I-labelled OC 125 monoclonal antibody F(ab')$_2$ fragments is insufficiently specific to be used as a screening test for endometriosis[6,7]. In a study of 28 women[7], immunoscintigraphy was positive in 22 women (16 with endometriosis, two with pelvic adhesions, one with pelvic inflammatory disease and one with normal pelvic findings) (Figures 4.19–4.24). Immunoscintigraphy was negative in five women (two with endometriosis and three with normal pelvic findings). One woman developed a hypersensitivity reaction and therefore did not receive the radiolabelled fragments.

(a)

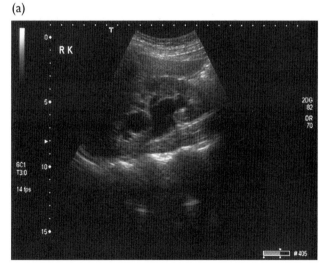

(b)

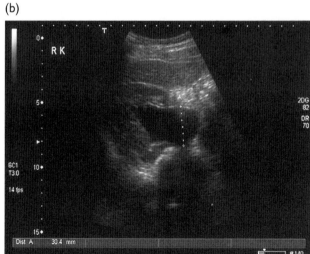

Figure 4.17 (a, b) Ultrasound images demonstrating hydroureter

(a)

(b)

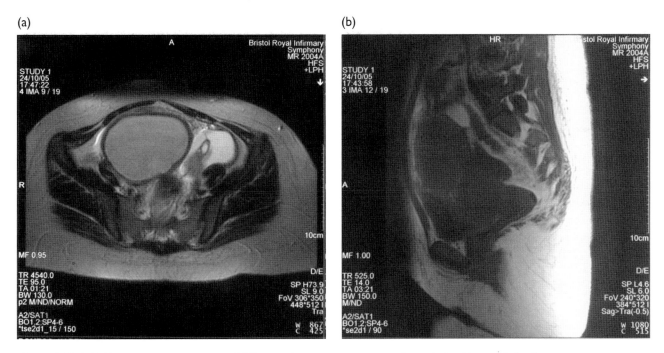

Figure 4.18 (a, b) Magnetic resonance imaging (MRI) scans demonstrating severe endometriosis with ureteric involvement

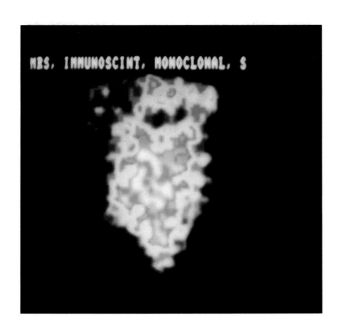

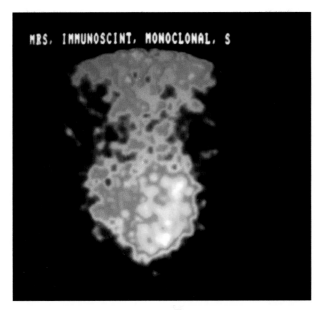

Figure 4.19 Posterior immunoscintigraphy view showing increased uptake in the right pelvis. Endometriosis was confirmed at operation and histologically. (Courtesy of Dr Basil Shepstone)

Figure 4.20 Anterior immunoscintigraphy view of the same patient as in Figure 4.19. There is increased uptake in the right pelvis. Endometriosis was confirmed at operation and histologically. (Courtesy of Dr Basil Shepstone)

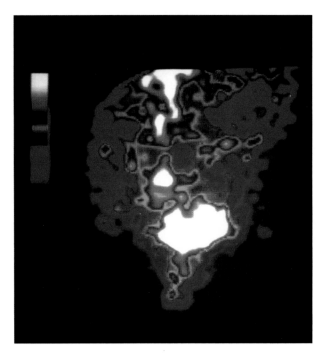

Figure 4.21 Anterior immunoscintigraphy view showing increased uptake in the pelvis, with more uptake on the left. Chocolate cysts were removed from both ovaries at laparotomy. Histology confirmed a right ovarian endometrioma, but only organising blood clot and compressed glands in the left ovary. (Courtesy of Dr Basil Shepstone)

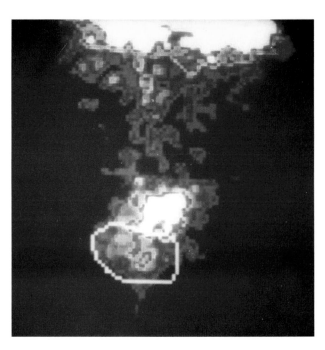

Figure 4.23 Posterior immunoscintigraphy view of the same patient as in Figures 4.21 and 4.22. (Courtesy of Dr Basil Shepstone)

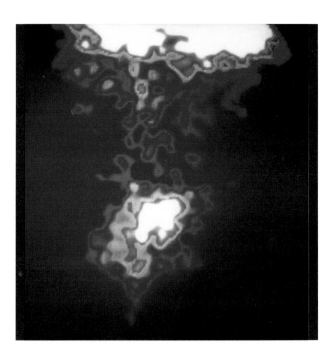

Figure 4.24 Posterior immunoscintigraphy view of the same patient as in Figures 4.21–4.23. (Courtesy of Dr Basil Shepstone)

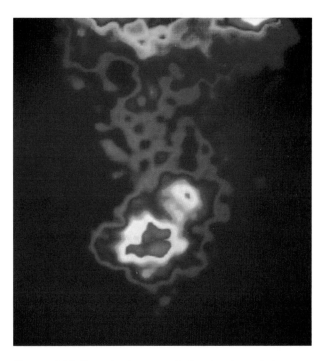

Figure 4.22 Posterior immunoscintigraphy view of the same patient as in Figure 4.21. There is increased uptake in the pelvis, with more uptake on the left. Chocolate cysts were removed from both ovaries at laparotomy. Histology confirmed a right ovarian endometrioma, but only organising blood clot and compressed glands in the left ovary. (Courtesy of Dr Basil Shepstone)

REFERENCES

1. Barbieri RL. CA-125 in patients with endometriosis. Fertil Steril 1986; 45: 767–9.

2. Mol BW, Bayram N, Lijmer JG, et al. The performance of CA-125 measurement in the detection of endometriosis: a meta-analysis. Fertil Steril 1998; 70: 1101–8.

3. Acien P, Shaw RW, Irvine L, Burford G, Gardner RL. CA 125 levels in endometriosis patients before, during and after treatment with danazol or LHRH agonists. Eur J Obstet Gynecol Reprod Biol 1989; 32: 241–6.

4. Moore J, Copley S, Morris J et al. A systematic review of the accuracy of ultrasound in the diagnosis of endometriosis. Ultrasound Obstet Gynecol 2002; 20: 630–4.

5. Kinkel K, Chapron C, Balleyguier C et al. Magnetic resonance imaging characteristics of deep endometriosis. Hum Reprod 1999; 14: 1080–6.

6. Kennedy SH, Soper ND, Mojiminiyi OA, Shepston BJ, Barlow DH. Immunoscintigraphy of ovarian endometriosis. A preliminary study. Br J Obstet Gynaecol 1988; 95: 693–7.

7. Kennedy SH, Mojiminiyi OA, Soper ND, Shepstone BJ, Barlow DH. Immunoscintigraphy of endometriosis. Br J Obstet Gynaecol 1990; 97: 667–70.

CHAPTER 5

Classification and histological diagnosis

CLINICAL CLASSIFICATION

The extent of endometriosis is usually staged by the American Fertility Society (AFS) classification system[1–3]. Four anatomical areas (peritoneum, fallopian tubes, ovaries and pouch of Douglas) are examined for the presence of endometriosis or adhesions. It evaluates the sequelae of endometriosis in terms of fibrosis, adhesions or cyst formation, but not the implants in terms of cells or evolution[4]. This system was devised to evaluate the results of surgical treatment. The high scores achieved in the presence of adhesions mean that endometriosis is classified as moderate or severe, even though the active disease process may have been eliminated and only the adhesions persist. What is called stage I or minimal endometriosis may represent a pelvis full of active, atypical endometriosis as well as a single inactive healed implant.

The development of a clinically useful classification system of endometriosis requires an understanding of the natural development and pathophysiology of the disease. The pathophysiology of endometriosis may change during its evolution. A more functional classification system of endometriosis is needed. Implants have been found to differ in their functional activity, with red petechial implants producing the highest amount of prostaglandin, brown producing less and black implants producing the least[5]. Free endometrial implants may be more related to infertility, and active enclosed implants to pelvic pain.

The existing classification correlates well with the chance of spontaneous conception. Women with minimal–mild endometriosis have near normal conception rates, while women with moderate and severe disease have reduced conception rates. The classification is deficient in its description for women with pain. Non-clinical information such as biochemical and endocrinological data, peritoneal fluid and blood markers as well as genetic information could also be included. The classification also needs to be expanded to describe women with retroperitoneal disease, deep peritoneal disease involving the bowel and adenomyosis.

A number of classification systems have been described. These include those by Acosta and colleagues[6], Kistner and co-workers[7] and the AFS classification system of 1979[1] and its modifications in 1985[2] and 1997[3]. Primarily, all divide endometriosis into various stages, with severity increasing with involvement of the ovaries and adhesion formation. All classification systems aim to try to correlate increasing severity of the disease with subsequent fertility outcome. However, for many women, the recurrent, long-standing nature of the disease is one of pain. This factor needs to be incorporated to try to achieve a classification scheme that may be predictive for pain and/or recurrence, rather than trying merely to predict fertility. A single classification incorporating all of these goals may be impossible. To date, the revised AFS system is used most commonly in investigative studies, and at least allows a comparison between the results published by different authors. This is illustrated in Figure 5.1.

In addition to the revised AFS score, it may be helpful to chart carefully the exact sites of all implants and their sizes, as used in the scheme of additive diameters of implants, described by Doberl and colleagues[8]. This gives a simple quantitative valuation of alteration in the 'volume' – although not the activity – of endometriotic disease following surgical or medical treatment.

Currently, endometriosis is diagnosed from both its typical and its atypical laparoscopic appearances and histological features. Both of these will be discussed below.

LAPAROSCOPIC APPEARANCES

The diagnosis of endometriosis requires visual assessment of the pelvis by laparotomy or laparoscopy. Deep and infiltrating endometriosis can be diagnosed by feel, using a blunt probe to assess whether a nodule is superficial or deep. As laparoscopic skills and techniques have developed, so more subtle appearances of endometriosis, such as nonpigmented implants, have been recognised[9]. In one study, the incidence of endometriosis rose due to increased recognition of 'subtle' implants from 15% of laparoscopies between January and May 1986 to 65% in the period October 1987 to June 1988[10].

AMERICAN SOCIETY FOR REPRODUCTIVE MEDICINE
REVISED CLASSIFICATION OF ENDOMETRIOSIS

Patient's Name _____ Date _____

Stage I   (Minimal)   - 1–5
Stage II   (Mild)   - 6–15
Stage III (Moderate) - 16–40
Stage IV (Severe)   - >40

Laparoscopy _____ Laparotomy _____ Photography _____

Recommended treatment _____

Total _____   Prognosis _____

PERITONEUM	ENDOMETRIOSIS		< 1 cm	1–3 cm	> 3 cm
		Superficial	1	2	4
		Deep	2	4	6
OVARY	R	Superficial	1	2	4
		Deep	4	16	20
	L	Superficial	1	2	4
		Deep	4	16	20
	POSTERIOR CUL-DE-SAC OBLITERATION		Partial		Complete
			4		40
	ADHESIONS		< 1/3 Enclosure	1/3–2/3 Enclosure	> 2/3 Enclosure
OVARY	R	Filmy	1	2	4
		Dense	4	8	16
	L	Filmy	1	2	4
		Dense	4	8	16
TUBE	R	Filmy	1	2	4
		Dense	4*	8*	16
	L	Filmy	1	2	4
		Dense	4*	8*	16

* If the fimbriated end of the Fallopian tube is completely enclosed, change the point assignment to 16

Denote appearance of superficial implant types as red ([R], red, red–pink, flamelike, vesicular blobs, clear vesicles), white ([W], opacifications, peritoneal defects, yellow–brown) or black ([B], black, hemosiderin deposits, blue). Denote percent of total described as R___%, W___% and B___%. Total should equal 100%.

Additional Endometriosis: _____ Associated Pathology: _____

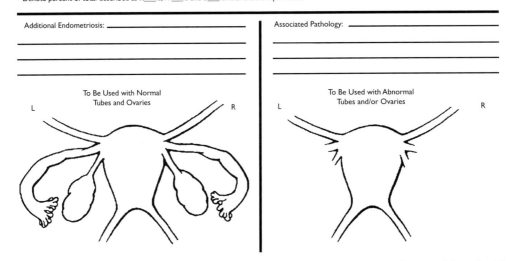

To Be Used with Normal Tubes and Ovaries

To Be Used with Abnormal Tubes and/or Ovaries

Figure 5.1 The American Society for Reproductive Medicine revised classification of endometriosis. (Reprinted from *Fertil Steril*, 67, Revised American Society for Reproductive Medicine classification of endometriosis: 1996, 817–21, © 1997, with permission from the American Society for Reproductive Medicine)

Laparoscopy is associated with significant morbidity, and it has a number of inherent faults. The diagnostic accuracy of laparoscopy relies upon the operator's visual and subjective assessment of the pelvis. The surgeon's experience, the presence of coexisting pelvic adhesions and preoperative bias can all influence the interpretation of the laparoscopic findings[11]. In addition, microscopic disease that has been described in visually normal peritoneum[12,13] can theoretically be missed at laparoscopy. Microscopic disease has been found in the visually normal peritoneum of 13% of women with and 6% without endometriosis[14] (this difference is not significant). However, Redwine[15] failed to demonstrate any endometriosis in biopsies from normal peritoneum taken from 33 women, of whom 24 had endometriosis elsewhere and nine had a normal pelvis at laparoscopy. He argued that the discrepancy between his and previous findings could only be explained by 'the discriminatory threshold of the clinicians' in defining what is visually normal peritoneum.

HISTOLOGICAL CLASSIFICATION

Types of implant

More than 15 laparoscopic appearances of peritoneal endometriosis have been described (Table 5.1). The classical implant is a nodular implant characterised by a variable degree of fibrosis and pigmentation. The colour can vary from white to blue, brown or black. Implants may be vesicular (frequently red in appearance), papular (usually whitish or yellow) or haemorrhagic[9]. On histological examination, the biopsies of such implants show glandular tissue in 50–95% of biopsies[17]. Atypical appearances include areas of hypervascularisation, white opacification, glandular excrescences, red flame-like lesions, yellow-brown patches, circular peritoneal defects and subovarian adhesions. Histological examination of these implants has identified endometriotic elements in varying percentages of cases[9,10,19] (Table 5.2). Healed implants present as nodular or fibrotic scar tissue. The peritoneal implants may represent different stages of the disease and further studies are needed to clarify the evolution of these implants. Laparoscopic criteria to distinguish between active and inactive implants have not been established.

Classical implants

The classical implant is a nodular implant characterised by varying degrees of fibrosis and pigmentation, such that the colour may vary from white to brown or black. Brown and black colouration appears to be a function of the amount of intraluminal haemosiderin and debris present.

Histological examination of biopsies from such implants shows glandular tissue making up over 90% of the implant. Endometrial tissue is represented by glandular epithelium surrounded by stroma. The glandular epithelium shows varying degrees of activity, but is often inactive with no apparent changes during the menstrual cycle (Figures 5.2 and 5.3).

Vesicular implants

Vesicular implants are small (diameter less than 5 mm) and may occur singly or in clusters. These implants are characterised by prominent vascularisation and are frequently red in appearance. The surrounding peritoneum may also show increased vascularisation. The endometrial tissue shows the presence of surface epithelium covering a highly vascularised stroma. Fluid accumulates between the surface of the implant and the overlying peritoneum, resulting in a blister or vesicle/bleb formation (Figures 5.4 and 5.5).

White vesicular implants may also be seen when there is an absence of bleeding, and the vast majority have histologically proven endometriotic tissue. These implants may represent very early stages in the development of an implant before vascularisation has been established and haemorrhage ensues.

Papular implants

The papular implant is another small implant with a diameter of less than 5 mm and again occurs singly or in clusters (Figures 5.6 and 5.7). The colour of these implants is usually whitish or sometimes yellow. Histologically, cystic glandular structures with stroma are found enclosed in the subperitoneal tissue. The peritoneum overlying the implant is often vascularised, and an accumulation of secretory products results in a cystic structure containing whitish or yellow opaque fluid.

Haemorrhagic implants

The haemorrhagic implants develop when implants have a surface epithelium covered by stroma with a good vascular supply (Figures 5.8 and 5.9). Proliferation, secretion and vesicle formation occur with these implants, and they haemorrhage perimenstrually. Haemorrhagic implants are more active implants.

Table 5.1 Histological characteristics of endometriotic implants and their laparoscopic appearance[16]

Histological type	Laparoscopic appearance	Components	Hormonal response
Free	Hemorrhagic vesicles and blebs	Surface epithelium glands and stroma	Proliferative, secretory and menstrual
Enclosed	Papules and (later) nodules	Glands and stroma	Proliferative, variable secretory, no menstruation
Healed	White nodules or flattened fibrotic scars	Glands only	No response

Table 5.2 Histological examination of atypical implants[18]

Implant	Endometriotic elements
Classical	93%
White opacified	81%
Red flame-like	81%
Glandular	67%
Hypervascularisation	50%
Subovarian adhesions	50%
Yellow-brown patches	47%
Circular peritoneal defects	45%

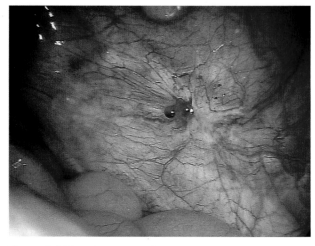

Figure 5.4 Vesicular implant of the ovarian fossa

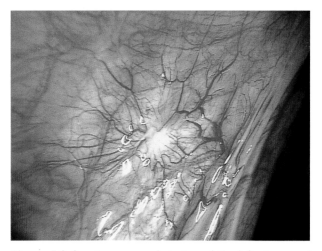

Figure 5.2 Scarring neovascularisation of the left uterosacral ligament

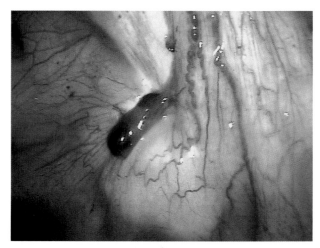

Figure 5.5 Vesicular implant below the right uterosacral ligament with tethering of the rectum

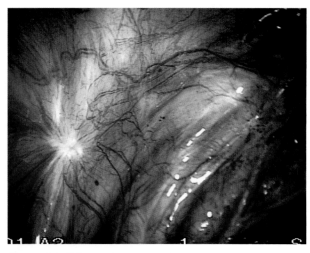

Figure 5.3 White endometriotic deposit with neovascularisation on the left uterosacral ligament

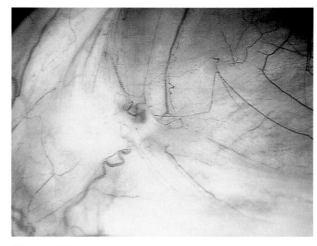

Figure 5.6 Papular implant on the pelvic side wall with fibrosis and neovascularisation

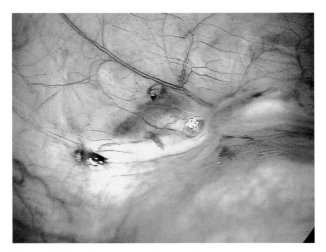

Figure 5.7 Papular implant with active haemorrhage

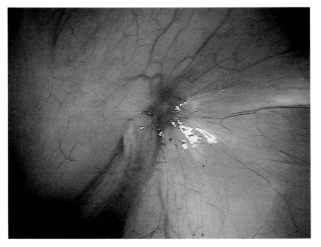

Figure 5.8 Haemorrhagic implant with haemosiderin staining

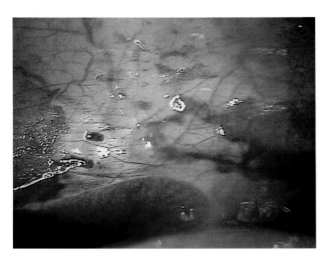

Figure 5.9 Haemosiderin staining and hypervascularisation

Nodular implants

Papular, nodular implants have no surface epithelium, and their components show cyclical proliferation and vasodilatation only and usually do not reach full secretory activity. There is no menstrual bleeding within the implants.

Healed implants

Healed implants may still contain cystic glands, but these are scant and there is no stroma. The healed implants are surrounded by connective tissue and present as nodular or fibrotic scarred areas.

Three-dimensional architecture of endometriosis

The three-dimensional evaluation of peritoneal endometriosis (Figure 5.10) has demonstrated two different types of peritoneal endometrial lesions, according to the degree of ramification[20]. The first type is composed of

(a)

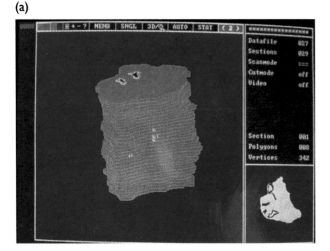

(b)

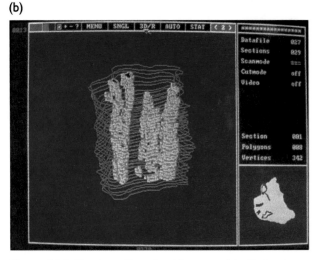

Figure 5.10 The three-dimensional image models displayed as a transparent structure. The stromal, epithelial and luminal structures are simultaneously shown: (a) indicated as a solid structure, (b) indicated as a transparent structure. (Reproduced from reference 20, with permission)

cylinder-like glands without ramifications. The second type is composed of ramified and connected glands. The distribution of glandular structures in the stroma is irregular, and the luminal structures are interconnected. Stereometric evaluation demonstrates a higher vascularisation and mitotic activity in red lesions, and it was proposed that such lesions were the first stage of implantation[21]. The depth of infiltration of endometriotic lesions is also important. Deep endometriosis is active disease and often associated with pelvic pain[22].

EVOLUTION OF IMPLANTS

Colour and direct appearance are the important macroscopic features of endometriosis. Data have been published suggesting a correlation between the woman's age and the colour and type of implants visualised[23]. This study showed younger women (less than 25 years of age) to have more non-pigmented implants, whilst older women (over 30 years of age) tended to have more pigmented implants, as well as more advanced disease.

The early manifestations of the disease are the subtle or non-coloured lesions, such as white lesions (white opacification). The presence of lower mitotic activity and poor stromal vascularisation in white lesions suggests that this type of lesion is a quiescent form of the disease. Red lesions (red vesicles, polypoid lesions, flame-like lesions) are more active forms of the disease. It is proposed that red lesions are more aggressive and progress to the so-called typical or black lesions, which should be considered as an enclosed implant surrounded by fibrosis.

It is not uncommon to see many different types of implant within the same woman, and the varying appearances described may well represent changes in the evolution of the deposit (Table 5.3). Enclosed active implants may heal, depending on regression of the stromal component and increasing connective tissue fibrosis. Flattening and

evolutionary changes in the glandular epithelium are characteristic of a healed implant. Frequently, glandular tissue is not found in white fibrotic 'healed' implants.

The haemorrhagic vesicle is likely to develop into a white or opaque papular implant. Epithelial tufts in the active gland can form polypoidal structures emerging on the surface of the implant, producing the haemorrhagic vesicle. Vascularised polyps respond in a manner similar to superficial endometrium to ovarian hormones, resulting in vascular necrosis at the time of menstruation. These changes induce an inflammatory reaction and fibroreactive tissue in the surrounding tissues. Hence, these modify the free haemorrhagic implant, inducing a surface covering to the active implant. The implant may then either continue to grow and become a deep implant, leading possibly to infiltration, or, conversely, undergo spontaneous healing if hormonal and vascular support are reduced and fibrosis predominates.

OVARIAN ENDOMETRIOSIS

In the ovary, endometriosis presents either as superficial haemorrhagic implants or in the more severe form as a haemorrhagic or 'chocolate' cyst (Figures 5.11 and 5.12). The histopathology of ovarian endometriosis is characterised by a large variation in the amount of endometrial tissue. The endometrial cyst can be lined by free endometrial tissue, histologically and functionally indistinguishable from eutopic endometrium, or all traces of endometrial tissue can be lost and the cyst wall covered by fibrotic and reactive tissue (Figures 5.13–5.15). No specific pathology can be found in up to one-third of clinically typical endometriosis cases, and these cysts are classified as haemorrhagic cysts (compatible with endometriosis). Both types of ovarian endometriosis are associated commonly with adhesion formation, and endometriosis should be suspected clinically if the ovary is adherent to the ovarian fossa.

Table 5.3 Frequency of location of endometriotic implants in the pelvis (from review of 500 consecutive cases, many women having multiple sites of involvement)

Site	Percentage
Uterosacral ligaments	63
Ovary superficial	56
Ovary deep (endometrioma)	19.5
Ovarian fossae	32.5
Anterior vesical pouch	21.5
Pouch of Douglas	18.5
Broad ligament	7.5
Intestines	5
Fallopian tube/mesosalpinx	4
Salpingitis isthmica nodosa	3
Uterus	4.5

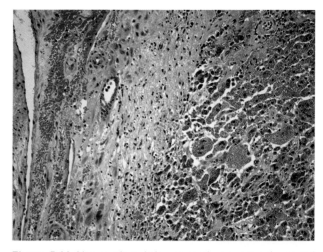

Figure 5.11 Haemosiderin-laden macrophages giving the typical brown appearance of a chocolate cyst. (Courtesy of Dr Joya Pawade)

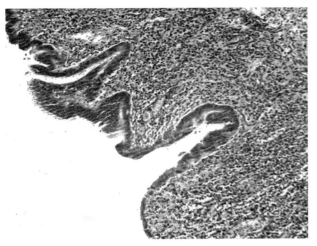

Figure 5.12 Haemorrhagic endometriotic cyst. (Courtesy of Dr Joya Pawade)

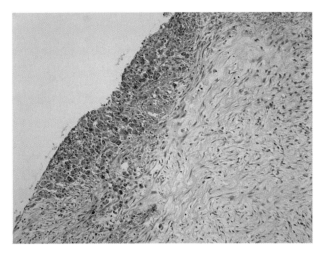

Figure 5.15 Lining is predominantly haemosiderin-laden macrophages typical of an endometriotic cyst. (Courtesy of Dr Joya Pawade)

RECTOVAGINAL ENDOMETRIOSIS

There is evidence that rectovaginal endometriosis differs morphologically and histologically from peritoneal endometriosis[24]. It is proposed that the rectovaginal adenomyotic nodule is a specific disease, different from peritoneal endometriosis. Mitotic activity, stromal vascularization and the epithelium/stroma ratio are all significantly different in peritoneal and rectovaginal endometriosis. Glandular epithelium predominates in rectovaginal nodules where stroma is sometimes absent.

It has been difficult to develop visual criteria for distinguishing deep infiltration from superficial disease by observation of the surface at laparoscopy. Infiltrating endometriosis (adenomyoma) and the difficulties it presents were noted by Sampson in 1921[25]. In these deep implants, there is a combination of varying amounts of fibromuscular scar and the glands and stroma of endometriosis (Figures 5.16–5.18). The degree of penetration can vary from as little as 2–3 mm in the majority of implants to more than 5 mm in 25% of implants. Infiltrating, deep implants may be easier to palpate than to see laparoscopically.

Koninckx[26] described three types of deeply infiltrating endometriosis: type I is a rather large lesion in the peritoneal cavity, infiltrating conically with the deeper parts becoming progressively smaller; type II has the main feature of the bowel being retracted over the lesion, which thus becomes deeply situated in the rectovaginal septum although not actually infiltrating it; and type III lesions are the deepest and most severe. They are spherically shaped, situated deep in the rectovaginal septum, often only visible as a small typical lesion at laparoscopy or often not visible at all. This lesion is often more palpable than visible, and is acutely tender if the patient is examined at the time of menstruation, and gives rise to dyspareunia.

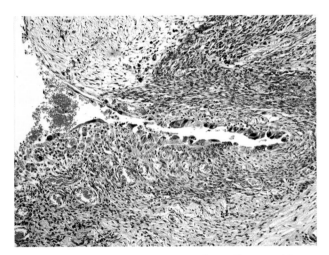

Figure 5.13 Haemosiderin-laden macrophages, fibrosis and haemorrhage. (Courtesy of Dr Joya Pawade)

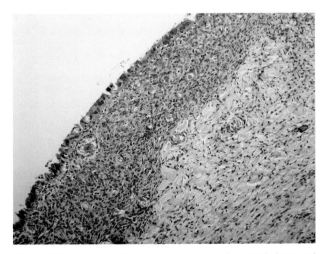

Figure 5.14 Endometriotic cyst showing surface epithelium and stroma. In the background there is contrasting ovarian stroma. (Courtesy of Dr Joya Pawade)

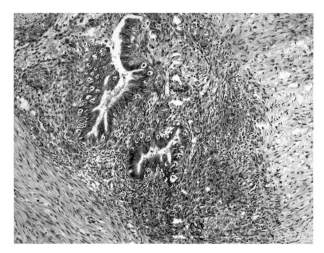

Figure 5.16 Deep local deposits within the parametrium showing glands and stroma. (Courtesy of Dr Joya Pawade)

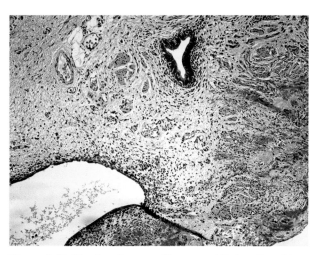

Figure 5.17 Glands and stroma. (Courtesy of Dr Joya Pawade)

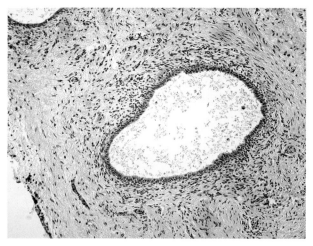

Figure 5.18 Deep endometriosis showing glandular structure and little surrounding stroma, found in 10% of women. (Courtesy of Dr Joya Pawade)

After gonadotropin-releasing hormone agonist treatment, active endometriosis and mitotic activity were significantly less in peritoneal, but not in rectovaginal endometriosis. It is proposed that some implants do not respond to hormonal treatment because (1) surrounding fibrosis prevents the drug from gaining access; (2) endometriotic cells have their own genetic programming, and endocrine influence is only secondary and dependent on the degree of differentiation of the cell; or (3) there are fewer oestrogen receptors, or the steroid receptors present are biologically inactive.

REFERENCES

1. American Fertility Society. Classification of endometriosis. Fertil Steril 1979; 32: 633–4.

2. American Fertility Society. Revised American Fertility Society classification of endometriosis: 1985. Fertil Steril 1985; 43: 351–2.

3. American Society for Reproductive Medicine. Revised American Society for Reproductive Medicine classification of endometriosis: 1996. Fertil Steril 1997; 67: 817–21.

4. Brosens IA, Cornillie F, Koninckx P, Vasquez G. Evolution of the revised American Fertility Society classification of endometriosis [Letter]. Fertil Steril 1985; 44: 714–16.

5. Vernon MW, Beard JS, Graves K, Wilson EA. Classification of endometriotic implants by morphologic appearance and capacity to synthesize prostaglandin. Fertil Steril 1986; 46: 801–6.

6. Acosta AA, Buttram VC, Besch PK, et al. A proposed classification of endometriosis. Obstet Gynecol 1973; 42: 19–25.

7. Kistner RW, Siegler AM, Behrman SJ. Suggested classification for endometriosis: relationship to infertility. Fertil Steril 1977; 28: 1008–10.

8. Doberl A, Bergquist A, Jeppson S et al. Repression of endometriosis following shorter treatment with or lower dose of danazol. Acta Obstet Gynecol Scand 1984; 123 (Suppl): 51–8.

9. Jansen RP, Russell P. Nonpigmented endometriosis: clinical, laparoscopic and pathologic definition. Am J Obstet Gynecol 1986; 155: 1154–9.

10. Martin DC, Hubert GD, van der Zwaag R, el-Zeky FA. Laparoscopic appearances of peritoneal endometriosis. Fertil Steril 1989; 51: 63–7.

11. Dmowski WP. Visual assessment of peritoneal implants for staging endometriosis: do number and cumulative size of implants reflect the severity of a systemic disease? Fertil Steril 1987; 47: 382–4.

12. Murphy AA, Green WR, Bobbie D, de la Cruz ZC, Rock JA. Unsuspected endometriosis documented by scanning electron microscopy in visually normal peritoneum. Fertil Steril 1986; 46: 522–4.

13. Vasquez G, Cornillie F, Brosens IO. Peritoneal endometriosis: scanning electron microscopy and histology of minimal pelvic endometriotic implants. Fertil Steril 1984; 42: 696–703.

14. Stripling MC, Martin DC, Chatman DL, van der Zwaag R, Poston WM. Subtle appearance of endometriosis. Fertil Steril 1988; 49: 427–31.

15. Redwine DB. Is 'microscopic' peritoneal endometriosis invisible? Fertil Steril 1988; 50: 665–6.

16. Brosens IA. The endometriotic implant. In: Thomas E, Rock J, eds. Modern Approaches to Endometriosis. Kluwer Academic, 1991: 21.

17. Nisolle M, Paindaveine B, Bourdon A et al. Histological diagnosis of peritoneal endometriosis in infertile women. Fertil Steril 1990; 53: 984–8.

18. Jansen RP, Russell P. Nonpigmented endometriosis: clinical, laparoscopic, and pathologic definition. Am J Obstet Gynecol 1986; 155: 1154–9.

19. Redwine DB. Age related evolution in color appearance of endometriosis. Fertil Steril 1987; 47: 1062–3.

20. Donnez J, Nisolle M, Casanas-Rouz F. Three-dimensional architectures of peritoneal endometriosis. Fertil Steril 1992; 57: 980–3.

21. Donnez J, Nisolle M, Casanas-Roux F. Peritoneal endometriosis: two-dimensional and three-dimensional evaluation of typical and subtle lesions. Ann NY Acad Sci 1994; 734: 342–51.

22. Koninckx PR, Martin D. Deep endometriosis: a consequence of deep infiltration or retraction or possible adenomyosis externa? Fertil Steril 1992; 58: 924–8.

23. Redwine DB. The distribution of endometriosis in the pelvis by age groups and fertility. Fertil Steril 1987; 47: 173–5.

24. Donnez J, Nisolle M, Casanas-Roux F, Brion P, Da Costa Ferreira N. Stereometric evaluation of peritoneal endometriosis and endometriotic nodules of the rectovaginal septum. Hum Reprod 1995; 11: 224–8.

25. Sampson JA. Perforating hemorrhagic (chocolate) cysts of the ovary, their importance and especially their relation to pelvic adenomas of endometrial type. Arch Surg 1921; 3: 245–323.

26. Koninckx PR. Deeply infiltrating endometriosis. In: Brosens I, Donnez J, eds. Endometriosis: Research and Management. Carnforth, UK: Parthenon Publishing, 1993: 437–46.

CHAPTER 6

Ovarian endometriosis

In the ovary, endometriosis presents either as superficial haemorrhagic implants or in the more severe form as a haemorrhagic or 'chocolate' cyst. The histopathology of ovarian endometriosis is characterised by a large variation in the amount of endometrial tissue. The endometrial cyst can be lined by free endometrial tissue, histologically and functionally indistinguishable from eutopic endometrium, or all traces of endometrial tissue can be lost and the cyst wall covered by fibrotic and reactive tissue. No specific pathology can be found in up to one-third of clinically typical endometriosis cases, and these cysts are classified as haemorrhagic cysts (compatible with endometriosis). Both types of ovarian endometriosis are associated commonly with adhesion formation and endometriosis should be suspected clinically if the ovary is adherent to the ovarian fossa (Figures 6.1 and 6.2).

SUPERFICIAL ENDOMETRIOSIS

Superficial implants can occur on all sides of the ovary, and can have varying and atypical appearances (Figures 6.3–6.6). Common superficial haemorrhagic implants are red vesicles or blebs, and the classical blue-black implants. Less common is the appearance of only yellowish-brown implants. Occasionally, there are clear papules, but it is essential that there should be other features of endometriosis present in the ovary before endometriosis is diagnosed, since these clear papules can very commonly be confused with Walthard's rests. Biopsy is advisable if other features of endometriosis are absent.

Haemorrhagic implants are commonly associated with adhesion formation, sometimes covering a significant proportion of the ovary. The adhesions can be difficult to detect by laparoscopy if they are avascular, transparent or in their early stages of development. This is particularly so when they are on the posterior aspect of the ovary. It is particularly important to examine all aspects of the ovary, so as not to miss the features of endometriosis. In the authors' opinion this would always involve the use of a second instrument to lift the ovary, rather than the practice of using the Veress needle.

ENDOMETRIOMA

The word 'endometrioma' is used to describe an endometriotic cyst of the ovary. Another term in widespread use is chocolate cyst, because of the characteristic dark brown or chocolate-coloured content of the cyst. Many haemorrhagic cysts are functional cysts, particularly corpus luteal cysts (Figure 6.7). The presence of other signs of endometriosis can help to distinguish between functional cysts and endometriosis.

In addition, aspiration of the chocolate content of the cyst can aid diagnosis (Figures 6.8 and 6.9). Other features, such as the site of the cyst on the lateral surface of the ovary, haemorrhagic adhesions and the puckering scar formation, indicate an endometriotic cyst. Haemorrhagic cysts of a different origin often contain large blood clots or even fresh haemorrhage, which is unlikely to be present with endometriosis. However, these characteristics can be lacking at laparoscopy, making it impossible to diagnose the endometriotic origin of the cyst without histological proof.

To aid diagnosis at laparoscopy, the cyst should be aspirated and the cyst cavity irrigated for direct observation of the wall. This commonly shows a uniform white fibrotic appearance but with hypervascularised, haemorrhagic foci in the more active cysts. The haemorrhagic content of the cyst is likely to originate from chronic bleeding from these small areas of free endometriosis.

FORMATION OF ENDOMETRIOMAS

It is thought that an endometrioma begins as an implant on the outer surface of the ovary. As it grows larger, the ovarian cortex becomes inverted, so that most endometriomas are attached to the outside of the ovary. Leakage from the cyst wall commonly leads to adhesion formation, particularly on the posterior surface of the ovary and in the ovarian fossa or to the posterior aspect of the broad ligament. Attempts to mobilise the ovary commonly result in rupture of the cyst and release of the contents. Adequate

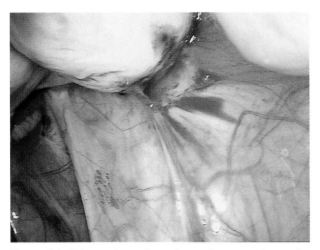

Figure 6.1 Right ovarian endometrioma adherent to the ovarian fossa

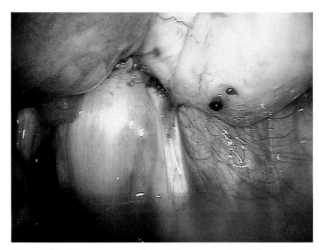

Figure 6.2 Close-up view of the right ovary and pouch of Douglas reveals superficial haemorrhagic vesicles on the right ovary and the extent of the adhesions

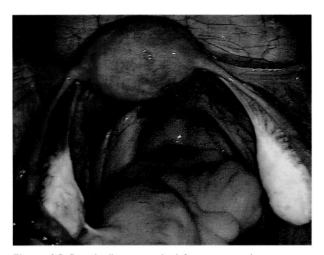

Figure 6.3 Bowel adherent to the left ovary secondary to superficial endometriosis

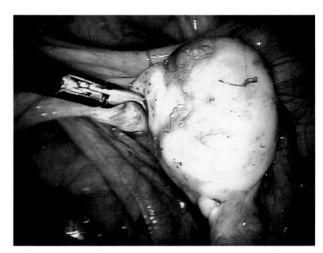

Figure 6.4 The ovary has been lifted up from the pelvic side wall revealing superficial endometriosis and haemosiderin staining

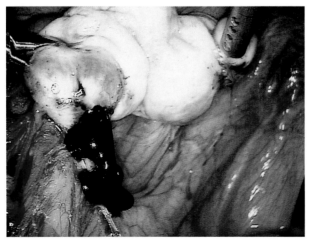

Figure 6.5 Left ovarian endometrioma

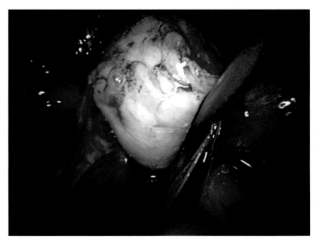

Figure 6.6 Superficial endometriosis of the ovary

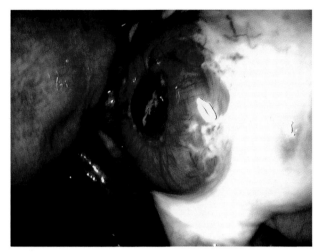

Figure 6.7 Corpus luteal cyst on the right ovary. The ovary was mobile with no evidence of endometriosis elsewhere

irrigation of the peritoneal cavity is necessary to remove all the cyst contents prior to closure (Figures 6.10 and 6.11).

In the treatment of ovarian endometriomas, it is essential that the cyst wall lining is completely excised or ablated to prevent recurrence.

SURGICAL TREATMENT OF ENDOMETRIOMAS

An endometrioma has typical features that make the macroscopic diagnosis very reliable[1]. These features include:

- size less than 12 cm in diameter
- adhesions to the pelvic side wall and/or posterior broad ligament
- 'powder burns' and minute red or black spots on the surface of the ovary
- tarry thick chocolate-coloured fluid content.

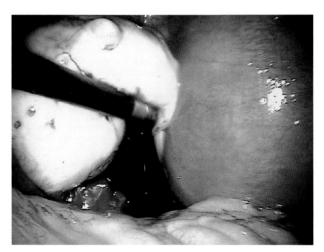

Figure 6.8 Left ovary adherent to the ovarian fossa. In releasing the ovary, the endometrioma has leaked

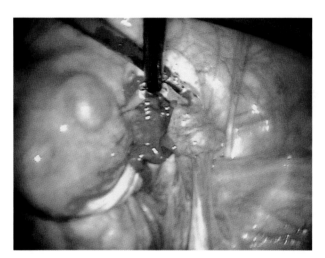

Figure 6.10 The leaking point is enlarged with scissors for formal ovarian cystectomy

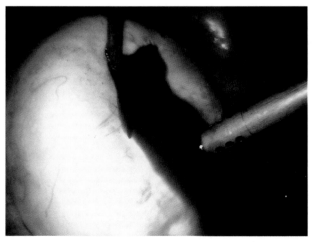

Figure 6.9 Aspiration and drainage of a left ovarian endometrioma

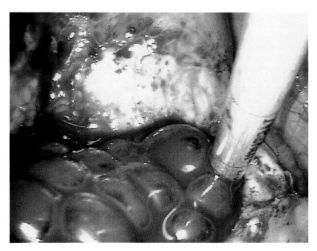

Figure 6.11 Aspiration of fluid in the pouch of Douglas

The removal of ovarian endometriomas can be difficult, as the capsule is often densely adherent. Large endometriomas are typically adherent to the back of the uterus or broad ligament or ovarian fossa (Figures 6.12 and 6.13). Adhesiolysis often results in opening of the cyst and leaking of the 'chocolate' content. This opening can be enlarged in order to carry out either formal cystectomy or laser photocoagulation and vaporisation of the cyst capsule. It is usually possible to remove a large cyst by stripping the capsule from the underlying ovarian stroma relatively easily, except at the invagination site where the capsule is densely adherent. Provided that there is haemostasis, the ovarian defect can be left open with little or no adhesion formation.

The surgical management of endometriomas was reviewed in the *Cochrane database of systematic reviews*[2]. No randomised studies of the surgical treatment of endometriomas by laparotomy were found. Two randomised trials of the laparoscopic treatment of ovarian endometriomas larger than 3 cm were included. Laparoscopic excision of the cyst wall was associated with a reduced rate of recurrence of endometriomas (odds ratio 0.41, confidence interval 0.18–0.93), reduced requirement for further surgery (odds ratio 0.21, confidence interval 0.05–0.79), reduced recurrence rates of the symptoms of dysmenorrhoea (odds ratio 0.15, confidence interval 0.06–0.38), dyspareunia (odds ratio 0.08, confidence interval 0.01–0.51) and non-menstrual pelvic pain (odds ratio 0.10, confidence interval 0.02–0.56). It was also associated with a subsequent increased rate of spontaneous pregnancy in women who had documented prior subfertility (odds ratio 5.21, confidence interval 2.04–13.29). The authors concluded that excisional surgery provided a more favourable outcome than drainage and ablation. However, no data as to the effect of either approach were found in women who subsequently underwent assisted reproductive techniques.

A general consensus is that ovarian endometriomas larger than 4 cm should be removed, both to reduce pain and to improve spontaneous conception rates. The presence of small endometriomas (2–4 cm) does not reduce the success of *in vitro* fertilisation (IVF) treatment[3]. However, there is an increased risk of developing a pelvic infection following transvaginal oocyte collection[4]. Expectant management without a tissue diagnosis does not exclude the possibility of malignancy, particularly in the older woman.

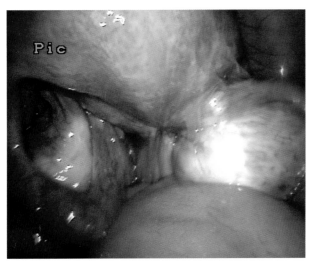

Figure 6.12 Bilateral endometriomas and tethering of the rectum

PATHWAY FOR MANAGEMENT OF THE ENDOMETRIOMA: RISK OF MALIGNANCY SCORING SYSTEM

The risk of malignancy is the ultrasound score multiplied by the menopausal score multiplied by the CA 125 level[5]. Since endometriosis is predominantly a disease of premenopausal women, the majority of women with an endometrioma will score less than 200. Women with a risk of malignancy score greater than 200 should be referred to a gynaecological oncologist. When obvious metastatic disease has been identified by ultrasound these women should be referred to a gynaecological oncologist regardless of the risk of malignancy score (Table 6.1).

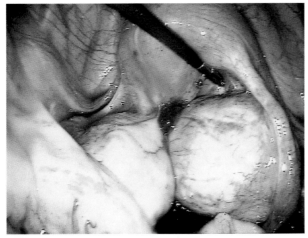

Figure 6.13 Bilateral ovarian endometriomas and 'kissing ovaries'

Table 6.1 The risk of malignancy index (RMI) scoring system

Feature	RMI score
Ultrasound features	0 = None
multilocular cyst	1 = One abnormality
solid areas	2 = Two or more
bilateral lesions	abnormalities
ascites	
intra-abdominal metastases	
Premenopausal	Score 1
Postmenopausal	Score 3
CA 125	Units/ml

POSSIBLE FUTURE TREATMENT

Ultrasound-guided aspiration of endometriomas leaving interleukin 2 in the cyst has been studied[6]. Nine of the 24 women who took part in the study required surgery within the follow-up period of 3 years.

REFERENCES

1. Vercellini P, Vendola N, Bocciolone L et al. Reliability of the visual diagnosis of ovarian endometriosis. Fertil Steril 1990; 53: 1198–200.

2. Hart RJ, Hickey M, Maouris P, Buckett W, Garry R. Excisional surgery versus ablative surgery for ovarian endometriomata. Cochrane Database Syst Rev 2005; (3): CD004992.

3. Tinkanen H, Kujansuu E. In vitro fertilisation in patients with ovarian endometriosis. Acta Obstet Gynecol Scand 2000; 79: 119–22.

4. Younis JS, Ezra Y, Laufer N, Ohel G. Later manifestation of pelvic abcesses following oocyte retrieval, for in vitro fertilization, in patients with severe endometriosis and ovarian endometrioma. J Assist Reprod Genet 1997; 14: 343–6.

5. Scottish Intercollegiate Guidelines Network (SIGN). Epithelial ovarian cancer. SIGN publication no. 75. Edinburgh: SIGN, October 2003.

6. Acien P, Perez-Albert G, Quereda FJ et al. Treatment of endometriosis with transvaginal ultrasound-guided drainage under GnRH analogues and recombinant interleukin-2 left in the cysts. Gynecol Obstet Invest 2005; 60: 224–31.

CHAPTER 7

Principles of treatment

The treatment of endometriosis needs to be tailored to the individual woman depending on her symptoms, priorities and the stage of endometriosis. Clinicians should be open and honest about the limitations of current treatment and the likelihood of recurrence.

WHEN TO USE SURGICAL OR MEDICAL TREATMENT?

Medical treatment relies on hormonal manipulation of the ovarian cycle and exerts an effect by inducing amenorrhoea. All types of medical treatment, except analgesics, are effective in reducing endometriosis-associated pain, but their side-effect profile limits their long-term use and recurrence is common on discontinuation. Medical treatment does not improve fertility and is contraceptive. If fertility is the priority, conservative surgery is effective in reducing endometriosis-associated pelvic pain as well as improving the chance of pregnancy.

Medical treatment does not improve fertility

Medical treatment of endometriosis produces no improvement in pregnancy rates compared to expectant treatment. Medical treatment with danazol[1], buserelin[2], medroxyprogesterone acetate[1], and gestrinone[3] was no more effective than placebo or expectant management in improving pregnancy rates.

Perhaps most important of all, it has also been shown that complete elimination of endometriosis by medical treatment does not return fertility to normal[3].

Assisted reproduction appears to have an overall benefit for all stages of treatment. The treatment of choice will depend on the severity of endometriosis, the woman's age, duration of infertility, past reproductive performance and the presence of other infertility factors such as tubal blockage or male factor infertility.

Medical treatment is effective treatment for pain

Medical treatment, therefore, should be reserved for those women who need treatment for pain, or as a preparation for surgery.

Surgical treatment is effective in the treatment of pain and fertility

Surgical treatment improves pain, particularly for women with more severe endometriosis. It improves pelvic pain and deep dyspareunia. The benefits of surgery are temporary, and by 12 months almost half of the women had recurrence of their pain and needed further medical treatment[4].

The aim of surgical treatment is to destroy or excise endometriotic nodules and divide peritubal or periovarian adhesions, restoring normal anatomy where possible (Figure 7.1). Cystectomy of ovarian endometriomas improves spontaneous pregnancy rates and reduces pain. In addition it may improve the response to *in vitro* fertilisation (IVF). Drawbacks of surgery include postoperative adhesion formation and incomplete removal of the disease.

PAIN

Sutton and colleagues randomly assigned 200 women to laparoscopic treatment or diagnostic laparoscopy[5]. Women who had laparoscopic treatment of endometriosis had less pain at 6 months' follow-up. Sixty-three women out of 100 in the treatment group and 23 of 100 in the diagnostic group had less pain. Looking at these results another way, 37 of the 100 women did not benefit in terms of pain. For women with very minimal endometriosis, 62 out of 100 women had no reduction in pain. Thus, surgery is more effective in reducing pain in women with more severe disease.

In a follow-up study[3], 44%, almost half of the treated women, had recurrence of pain requiring additional treatment, 1 year after surgery. Surgical failure may result from missed lesions, incomplete removal or recurrence of disease or because the pain was caused by something else (irritable bowel, for example). The results of surgery are temporary and as much deep disease as possible must be removed to achieve the best results (Figures 7.2 and 7.3).

FERTILITY

Surgical treatment of endometriosis results in a significant improvement in pregnancy rates. Surgical treatment of

(a)

(b)

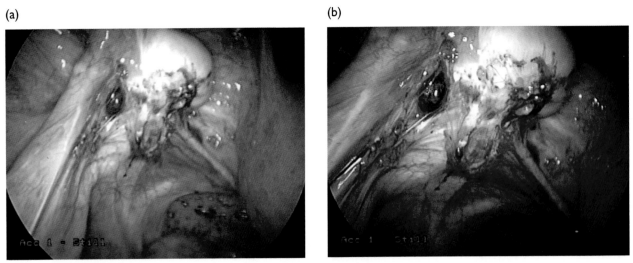

Figure 7.1 (a, b) Active endometriosis, periovarian adhesions resulting in tethering of the left ovary to pelvic side wall

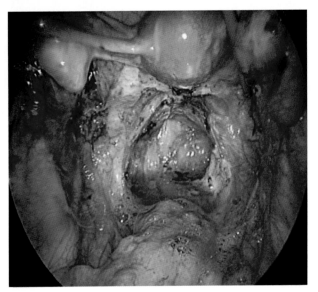

Figure 7.2 Completed dissection of the pouch of Douglas having excised deep rectovaginal deposits

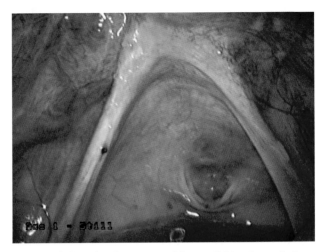

Figure 7.4 Stage I endometriosis with superficial endometriosis on the uterosacral ligament and peritoneal pocketing

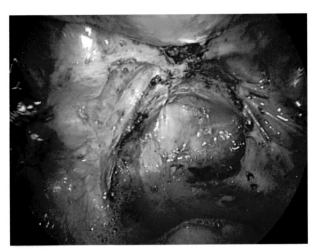

Figure 7.3 Close-up of the same view as shown in Figure 7.2

minimal to mild endometriosis improves the chance of pregnancy compared to diagnostic laparoscopy[6]. A total of 341 women with minimal–mild endometriosis were randomly assigned to treatment of endometriosis (excision, electrocautery or laser) or diagnostic laparoscopy. The different types of treatment all appeared equally effective. In the treated group, 50 of 172 (30%) became pregnant within 36 weeks compared to 29 of 169 (18%) in the diagnostic group. The miscarriage rate in both groups was 20% (Figures 7.4–7.7).

The Canadian study[6] was well designed, but criticisms were that the type of surgical treatment varied. Only the typical blue-black spots of endometriosis were included, and we now recognise many more appearances of the disease. Some women also had treatment of adhesions, which may have introduced bias. Some women were told what

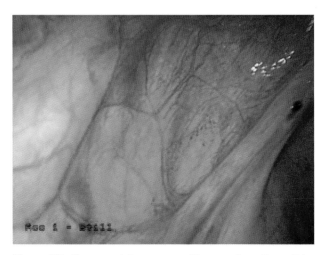

Figure 7.5 Close-up of the uterosacral ligament from Figure 7.4

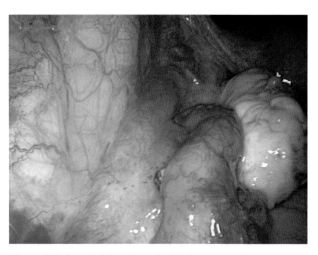

Figure 7.6 Superficial endometriosis, left ovary and tube

(a)

(b)

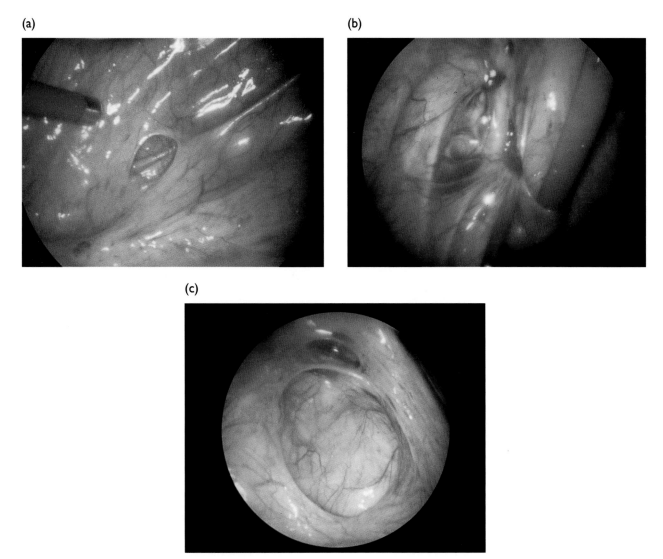

(c)

Figure 7.7 (a–c) Peritoneal pocketing in the pouch of Douglas with associated endometriosis

treatment they had had on discharge from hospital, which unblinded the trial. However, as a result of this study, it is reasonable to wait about a year following surgery before fertility treatment to see if natural conception will occur.

A smaller study produced conflicting results. The author found no difference between surgical treatment and diagnostic laparoscopy[7]. In the treated group, 10 of 51 (19.6%) and 10 of 45 (22.2%) in the control group became pregnant within 1 year following laparoscopy. It is possible that the lack of difference in this study was due to a lack of statistical power.

When the presenting symptom is pain, surgery is the treatment of choice in women with stage III and IV disease and may also improve fertility. Current opinion favours postoperative medical treatment for moderate–severe endometriosis, as this delays the recurrence of pelvic pain. IVF should be considered in these women, either as an alternative to surgery or following unsuccessful surgery.

Many studies have reported the poor outcome of IVF and embryo transfer in women with stage III and IV endometriosis compared to women with stage I and II endometriosis[8]. However, IVF with prolonged (2–7 months) down regulation using a long-acting gonadotropin releasing hormone (GnRH) agonist after surgical debulking results in good pregnancy rates, comparable to those achieved with other causes of infertility[9,10]. The presence of small endometriomas does not reduce the success of IVF treatment[11]. However, there is an increased risk of developing a pelvic infection following transvaginal oocyte collection[12].

PREVENTIVE TREATMENT

The combined oral contraceptive pill (COCP) has never been fully assessed in the treatment of endometriosis, particularly with pre- and post-treatment laparoscopy. However, in a comparative study, the COCP was as effective as a GnRH agonist in the treatment of pain associated with endometriosis[13].

COMBINED MEDICAL AND SURGICAL TREATMENT

Medical (drug) treatment after surgical treatment may delay the return of pain symptoms in a woman who does not wish to start trying to conceive immediately.

If surgery is to treat significant pain and a woman does not plan to have a family immediately, postoperative medical treatment has been shown to delay the return of symptoms. Different types of medical treatment all produce the same result. Research has shown that the COCP taken after surgery provides pain relief for up to 1 year after surgery[14].

ASSISTED REPRODUCTION

In vitro fertilisation can be considered as an alternative to surgery, particularly when pain is not severe, or following unsuccessful surgery.

There are several types of fertility treatment available. What type of fertility treatment depends on the severity of endometriosis, the woman's age, how long the couple have been trying to conceive, whether the couple have conceived in the past and other fertility factors such as blocked tube or sperm problems.

Ovarian stimulation with intrauterine insemination

Ovarian stimulation and intrauterine insemination (IUI) or superovulation and IUI aims to boost a woman's fertility so that she produces several eggs in one month (usually three or four). It is more effective than either no treatment or IUI alone in women who have not conceived naturally and who have minimal or mild endometriosis[15]. A live birth rate of 10–15% per treatment cycle can be expected. IUI is less expensive and less invasive than IVF or gamete intrafallopian transfer (GIFT) and should be considered initially in suitable patients. About 80% of couples who will conceive with IUI do so in the first 4–6 cycles. After three or four unsuccessful IUI treatment cycles, IVF or GIFT should be considered.

Gamete intrafallopian tube transfer (GIFT)

The oocytes are collected, inseminated with sperm and then both are transferred back to the fallopian tube before fertilisation takes place (Figures 7.8 and 7.9). GIFT is suitable for women with healthy fallopian tubes whose endometriosis is not severe; those who have failed to conceive by IUI; older women where the number of oocytes are fewer; women who have been trying to conceive for a long time; and couples with several factors causing infertility.

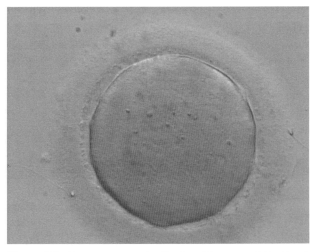

Figure 7.8 Oocyte prior to fertilisation. (Courtesy of Mr Alpesh Doshi)

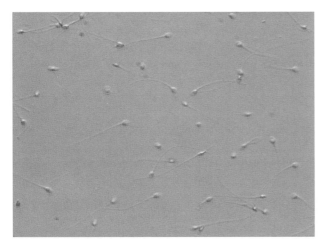

Figure 7.9 Spermatozoa. (Courtesy of Mr Alpesh Doshi)

In vitro fertilisation and embryo transfer

IVF and embryo transfer (Figrues 7.10–7.13) is an established and successful treatment for endometriosis-related infertility. IVF is suitable for women with damaged or blocked tubes; women with moderate or severe endometriosis; women with minimal or mild endometriosis with a partner who has sperm problems; and women who have failed to conceive by IUI.

Gonadotropin releasing hormone agonists have improved IVF success rates by reducing the numbers of cancelled cycles and preventing premature ovulation. Prolonged treatment with GnRH agonists results in a higher pregnancy rate[9,10]. Pregnancy and live birth rates are comparable to those with other causes of infertility. National data statistics quote a 22% live birth rate per IVF cycle started for women below the age of 38, and 19.5% for women of all ages[16]. This second figure is lower because age itself is a significant factor reducing female fertility.

The presence of small endometriotic ovarian cysts (endometriomas) does not decrease the success of IVF.

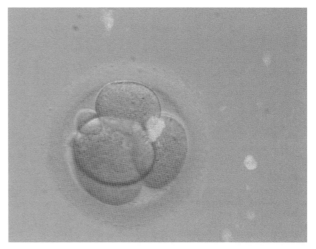

Figure 7.11 Four-cell embryo (day 2 after IVF). (Courtesy of Mr Alpesh Doshi)

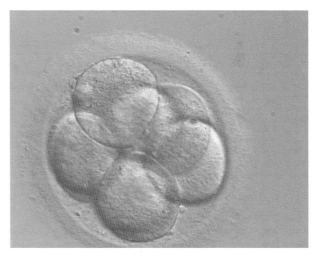

Figure 7.12 Eight-cell embryo (day 3 after IVF). (Courtesy of Mr Alpesh Doshi)

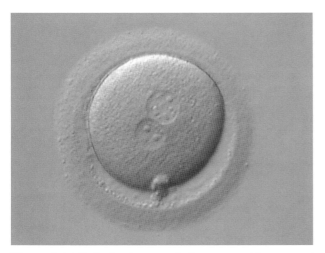

Figure 7.10 Early fertilisation of the oocyte. (Courtesy of Mr Alpesh Doshi)

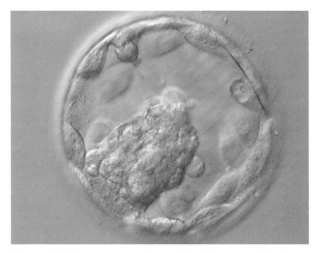

Figure 7.13 Blastocyst (day 5 after IVF). (Courtesy of Mr Alpesh Doshi)

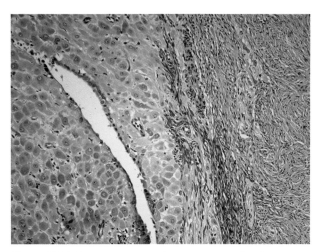

Figure 7.14 During pregnancy, the appearance of endometriosis changes. The epithelial glands appear inactive and the stroma are decidualised, compared to the background ovarian stroma. (Courtesy of Dr Joya Pawade)

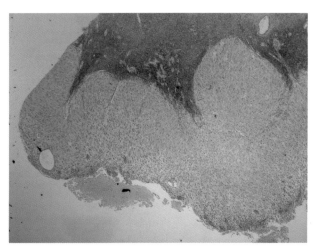

Figure 7.15 During pregnancy, the stroma becomes decidualised giving a dramatic and suspicious appearance macroscopically. (Courtesy of Dr Joya Pawade)

However, there is an increased risk of developing a pelvic infection following transvaginal egg (oocyte) collection[12]. It is generally suggested that endometriotic cysts over 5 cm in diameter are removed surgically prior to IVF.

Pregnancy and endometriosis

Endometriosis rarely causes problems during pregnancy (Figures 7.14 and 7.15). There are case reports of women whose pain has increased in the first few months of pregnancy. In general, pain improves, but is likely to recur at some point after delivery.

REFERENCES

1. Telimaa S. Danazol and medroxyprogesterone acetate inefficacious in the treatment of infertility in endometriosis. Fertil Steril 1988; 50: 872–5.

2. Mara R, Paielli FV, Muzil L, Dell'Acque S, Mancuso S. GnRH analogs versus expectant management in minimal-mild endometriosis-associated infertility. Acta Eur Fertil 1994; 25: 37–41.

3. Thomas EJ, Cooke ID. Successful treatment of asymptomatic endometriosis: does it benefit infertile women? Br Med J 1987; 294: 1117–19.

4. Sutton CJ, Pooley AS, Ewen SP, Haines P. Follow-up report on a randomised controlled trial of laser laparoscopy in the treatment of pelvic pain associated with minimal to moderate endometriosis. Fertil Steril 1997; 68: 1070–4.

5. Sutton CJ, Ewen S, Whitelaw N, Haines P. Prospective randomised, double-blind controlled trial of laser laparoscopy in the treatment of pelvic pain associated with minimal, mild and moderate endometriosis. Fertil Steril 1994; 62: 696–700.

6. Marcoux S, Maheux R, Berube S. Laparoscopic surgery in infertile women with minimal or mild endometriosis. Canadian Collaborative Group on Endometriosis. N Engl J Med 1997; 337: 217–22.

7. Parazzini F. Ablation of lesions or no treatment in minimal-mild endometriosis in infertile women: a randomized trial. Gruppo Italiano per lo studi dell'Endometriosi. Hum Reprod 1999; 14: 1332–4.

8. Azem F, Lessing JB, Geva E et al. Patients with stages III and IV endometriosis have a poorer outcome to in vitro fertilization-embryo transfer than patients with tubal infertility. Fertil Steril 1999; 72: 1107–9.

9. Nakamura K, Oosawa M, Kondou I et al. Menotropin stimulation after prolonged gonadotrophin releasing hormone agonist pretreatment for IVF in patients with endometriosis. J Assist Reprod Genet 1992; 9: 113–17.

10. Marcus SF, Edwards RG. High-rates of pregnancy after long-term down-regulation of women with severe endometriosis. Am J Obstet Gynecol 1994; 171: 812–17.

11. Tinkanen H, Kujansuu E. In vitro fertilisation in patients with ovarian endometriosis. Acta Obstett Gynecol Scand 2000; 79: 119–22.

12. Younis JS, Ezra Y, Laufer N, Ohel G. Later manifestation of pelvic abcesses following oocyte retrieval, for in vitro fertilization, in patients with severe endometriosis and ovarian endometrioma. J Assist Reprod Genet 1997; 14: 343–6.

13. Vercellini P, Trespidi L, Colombo A et al. A gonadotrophin releasing hormone agonist versus a low dose oral contraceptive for pelvic pain associated with endometriosis. Fertil Steril 1993; 60: 75–9.

14. Muzii L, Marana R, Caruana P et al. Postoperative administration of monophasic combined oral contraceptives after laparoscopic treatment of ovarian endometriomas: a prospective randomized trial. Am J Obstet Gynecol 2000; 183: 588–92.

15. Hughes EG. The effectiveness of ovulation induction and intrauterine insemination in the treatment of persistent infertility: a meta-analysis. Hum Reprod 1997; 12: 1865–72.

16. HFEA Guide to infertility – treatment and success data based on treatment carried out between 1 Apr 2003 and 31 Mar 2004. 2006–2007.

CHAPTER 8

Medical treatment of endometriosis

MEDICAL MANAGEMENT OF ENDOMETRIOSIS

Medical treatment is often first-line management treatment of pelvic pain (Table 8.1). It may also be used following surgery for endometriosis, either for recurrent pain, or prior to further definitive surgery. The choice of treatment is dictated by the age of the woman, family status, desire for conception, severity of symptoms, stage of disease and prior response to any treatment. In selecting the specific hormonal regimen, side-effects of the drug, individual sensitivity and response, as well as economic factors, may have to be considered.

NON-STEROIDAL ANTI-INFLAMMATORY DRUGS

Non-steroidal anti-inflammatory drugs do not treat endometriotic lesions but may be effective in the treatment of pelvic pain. In particular, the pain associated with dysmenorrhoea is mediated by prostaglandin synthesis[1]. Non-steroidal anti-inflammatory drugs inhibit cyclo-oxygenase and therefore reduce prostaglandin production and reduce pelvic pain.

The commonest non-steroidal anti-inflammatory drugs are ibuprofen and naproxen, which can be bought over the counter. Mefenamic acid is available on prescription only, and is effective in the treatment of dysmenorrhoea at a dose of 500 mg three times daily. The main side-effects are gastrointestinal, particularly gastric irritation. Peptic ulceration may result if treatment is used for a long period of time, although if taken for 5 days each month, it rarely causes a problem. A rare, but significant complication of long-term use is renal damage, resulting from capillary necrosis and ultimately renal failure.

Non-steroidal anti-inflammatory drugs were reviewed in the Cochrane database[2]. In the only randomised controlled trial of naproxen compared to placebo, there was no evidence of an effect on pain relief (odds ratio 3.27, 95% confidence interval 0.61–17.69) in women with endometriosis. There was also inconclusive evidence to indicate whether women taking non-steroidal anti-inflammatory drugs were less likely to require additional analgesia (odds ratio 0.12, 95% confidence interval 0.09–2.47) when compared to placebo.

A new generation of non-steroidal anti-inflammatory drugs, namely cyclo-oxygenase (COX)-2 inhibitors, have few gastrointestinal side-effects. They antagonise and prevent the effect of cyclo-oxygenase-2 and therefore have a much more specific effect on prostaglandin production. Selective COX-2 inhibitors, e.g. celecoxib/Celebrex®, rofecoxib/Vioxx®, valdecoxib/Bextra®, are similarly effective in treating pelvic pain or dysmenorrhoea[3], but considerably more expensive. Rofecoxib was recently withdrawn from the market because of myocardial infarction. It remains to be seen whether or not these new medications will replace conventional non-steroidal anti-inflammatory drugs as a first-line treatment.

THE ORAL CONTRACEPTIVE PILL

The oral contraceptive pill is often used as first-line treatment of endometriosis-associated pain. It may also be used empirically. The combined oral contraceptive (COC) pill reduces pain associated with endometriosis, is well tolerated and can be continued long-term for the control of symptoms. It is a safe and effective treatment for recurrent pelvic pain due to endometriosis. In healthy women without risk factors, the COC pill may be continued until the menopause.

The oral contraceptive pill mediates its effect by suppressing ovulation and creating a pseudopregnancy hormonal environment. It is effective in regulating the menstrual pattern, reducing menstrual blood loss and improving dysmenorrhoea. When taken daily on a continuous basis for three pill packets, amenorrhoea is likely to be induced and this regime is well tolerated.

In uncontrolled studies, the oral contraceptive pill is effective treatment for dysmenorrhoea[4]. In a controlled study comparing the combined oral contraceptive pill with gonadotropin releasing hormone agonist, the pill was as

Table 8.1 Medical treatments for endometriosis

Treatment	Mode of action	Side-effects
Progestogens	Decidualization followed by atrophy	Breakthrough bleeding, weight gain, bloating, acne, mood changes
Combined oral contraceptive pill	Suppression of ovulation Hypo-oestrogenic state	Weight gain, headache, nausea, breast enlargement, depression, risk of thromboembolism
Androgenic agents danazol	Suppression of hypothalamic–pituitary axis	Weight gain, acne, oily skin, muscle cramps, hot flushes, depression, hirsutes, skin rash, deepening of the voice
Androgenic agents gestrinone	Suppression of hypothalamic–pituitary axis	As for danazol but fewer side-effects
Gonadotropin releasing hormone agonists	Pituitary gonadotroph, desensitisation via downregulation of gonadotropin releasing hormone receptors	Hot flushes, headache, vaginal dryness, reduced libido

effective in the treatment of deep dyspareunia and non-cyclical pain[5]. A randomised trial in 57 women with pain and laparoscopically confirmed endometriosis, treated for 6 months with 20 mg ethinyl oestradiol plus desogestrel 150 mg or goserelin 3.6 mg every 28 days showed a reduction in pelvic pain and deep dyspareunia in both groups[5]. The incidence of side-effects was significantly reduced in the women taking the COC pill (Table 8.2). At 12 months, pain relief was continued, with no difference between the two groups.

A randomised controlled study demonstrated that the continuous monophasic oral contraceptive pill was also an effective, safe and inexpensive treatment for recurrent pelvic pain due to endometriosis[6].

GESTOGENS AND ANTIGESTOGENS

Progestins

Progestins are an important treatment option in the management of endometriosis-associated pain. Oral Provera® 50 mg daily is an effective treatment regimen, although some women will not tolerate it due to the side-effects.

Subjective improvement in pain has been reported with several of the progestogens. The larger progestogen studies have involved the use of medroxyprogesterone acetate (MPA) at a dose of 30–50 mg[7–9]. These have been open studies,

Table 8.2 The incidence of side-effects was significantly reduced in women taking the combined oral contraceptive (COC) pill compared to those taking gonadotropin releasing hormone agonist (GnRHa)[5]

	GnRHa	COC pill
Hot flushes	83%	4%
Insomnia	24%	0%
Vaginal dryness	17%	0%

but each has reported good relief of symptoms, and in one controlled study, MPA 100 mg daily was found to have equivalent efficacy to danazol 600 mg daily with both drugs performing significantly better than placebo in the relief of pelvic pain[10].

Progestins exert their effect by causing pseudodecidualisation followed by atrophy of both endometrium and endometriosis. Amenorrhoea results in an improvement in dysmenorrhoea and pelvic pain, with high patient satisfaction rates[7]. Possible side-effects include water retention, weight gain and irregular vaginal bleeding.

Depo-Provera®

Intramuscular Depo-Provera® is an alternative to oral medroxyprogesterone acetate. It is more often used for contraception, but has been shown to be effective in inducing amenorrhoea and improving endometriosis-associated pelvic pain. Depo-Provera is as effective as low-dose danazol combined with an oral contraceptive pill, but has far fewer side-effects[11]. The major side-effects of Depo-Provera include weight gain, breast tenderness. There may be prolonged amenorrhoea following termination of treatment. It is this last side-effect that limits use for women wishing to seek fertility in the short term.

Published in 1996, depot medroxyprogesterone acetate was as effective as leuprorelide in the reduction of endometriosis-associated pain[12]. Some 300 women with laparoscopically proven endometriosis were randomly assigned to 6 months' treatment with either subcutaneous injection of 104 mg depot medroxyprogesterone acetate every 3 months or leuprorelide 3.75 mg monthly or 11.25 mg every 3 months, with 12 months' post-treatment follow-up. Both treatments resulted in significant improvements in pain score. At 6 months, bone loss was significantly less with depot medroxyprogesterone acetate than with leuprorelide. Bone density had returned to normal by 12 months in the depot medroxyprogesterone acetate group, but not in the leuprorelide group.

The intrauterine progestogen only system

The levonorgestrel-releasing intrauterine system (Mirena® IUS) significantly reduces menstrual blood flow and dysmenorrhoea in women with endometriosis[13,14]. The results of a small observational study demonstrated few side-effects and high satisfaction. Twenty women with recurrent moderate or severe dysmenorrhoea after conservative surgery for endometriosis had a levonorgestrel-releasing intrauterine system inserted[14]. Fifteen out of the 20 women had significantly reduced menstrual pain and amenorrhoea or hypomenorrhoea. Three were dissatisfied, and two were uncertain about whether the device had improved their symptoms.

Published in 2005, a randomised controlled trial compared the levonorgestrel-releasing intrauterine system with depot gonadotropin releasing hormone agonist for endometriosis-associated pain[15]. Eighty-two women were randomised to treatment. Both were effective in the treatment of pelvic pain associated with endometriosis, with no differences observed between the two treatments. Improvement was noticed as early as 1 month into treatment. Women with more severe endometriosis (stage III–IV) showed a more rapid improvement than women with milder disease (stage I–II). Bleeding was more common with the levonorgestrel-releasing hormone intrauterine system.

Cerazette®

Recently introduced as a progestogen-only contraceptive pill, Cerazette® contains levonorgestrel. It is more effective than other progestogen-only pills in preventing ovulation. The authors have used it with some success in the treatment of endometriosis-associated pain in women who are unable to tolerate or have contraindications for the combined oral contraceptive pill.

Danazol

Danazol is a synthetic derivative of 17-ethinyl testosterone and inhibits pituitary gonadotropin production and ovarian steroid release. This results in the suppression of ovulation and atrophy of the endometrium and endometriotic implants. In placebo-controlled studies, danazol at a dose of 600 mg per day improved endometriosis-associated pelvic pain[10]. It has both hypo-oestrogenic and androgenic side-effects. These include hot flushes, breakthrough bleeding, acne, hirsutes, muscle cramps and a reduction in breast size. Side effects are fewer at lower doses, but efficacy is reduced.

Given its side-effect profile and with alternative treatment available, danazol is now rarely used. It can, however, be extremely effective, and the authors know women who feel fantastically well on danazol and even refuse to discontinue treatment!

Gestrinone

Gestrinone is derived from 19-nortestosterone and causes endometrial and endometriosis atrophy. Similar to danazol, it reduces serum progesterone and has marked androgenic side-effects including acne and hirsuitism, as well as a negative effect on the lipid profile. At a dose of 2.5 mg weekly it has been shown to be effective in reducing pelvic pain. However, its side-effect profile limits its use.

GONADOTROPIN RELEASING HORMONE AGONISTS

Gonadotropin releasing hormone agonists induce, stimulate and bind to the gonadotropin receptors on the anterior pituitary resulting in downregulation and a hypo-oestrogenic state. Following initial stimulation of the anterior pituitary and a 'flare' of gonadotropin release, gonadotropin levels are suppressed and the ovaries become inactive with resulting amenorrhoea.

There are three modes of administration for the different types of gonadotropin releasing hormone agonist, dependent upon their half-life profile. Goserelin acetate (Zoladex®), leuprorelin acetate (Prostap®) and triptorelin (Decapeptyl® and Gonapeptyl Depot®) are subcutaneous or intramuscular injections. Buserelin (Suprefact®) and naferelin (Synarel®) are nasal sprays.

Placebo-controlled studies have reported a significant reduction in pelvic pain and dysmenorrhoea in women treated with gonadotropin releasing hormone agonists compared to placebo[16,17]. The majority of women on placebo discontinued treatment because of continuing pain.

The main side-effects of gonadotropin releasing hormone agonists are the significant hypo-oestrogenic symptoms such as hot flushes, night sweats, mood changes, sleep disturbance and vaginal dryness. In addition, 6 months' treatment results in a 3–5% loss in bone mineral density, which is at least partially reversible on cessation of treatment. Treatment is licensed for 6 months, although combined with add-back hormone replacement therapy, it has been continued for much longer.

A large number of open studies have shown that gonadotropin releasing hormone agonists reduce pain, and several randomised trials have compared gonadotropin releasing hormone agonists with danazol[18,19]. Six months' treatment with gonadotropin releasing hormone agonists significantly reduces pain, and this reduction is noted as early as the second month of treatment. This reduction in pain is maintained after stopping treatment, and 6 months later pain is still reduced compared to baseline. Neither treatment is superior for the relief of pain, and they differ only in their side-effect profile. A gonadotropin releasing hormone agonist has also been shown to be effective as a short-term first-line treatment for women with chronic pelvic pain prior to laparoscopy[20].

Gonadotropin releasing hormone agonists with add-back therapy

Gonadotropin releasing hormone agonist treatment is limited by the hypo-oestrogenic side-effects and the 5–6% loss in bone density during treatment.

Add-back therapy is effective in attenuating bone loss and reducing hypo-oestrogenic side-effects, without reducing the beneficial effect on endometriosis-related pain. The premise upon which this is made is that low-dose oestrogen replacement is sufficient to alleviate the hypo-oestrogenic symptoms, but not high enough to stimulate the endometriosis. Combined oestrogen and progestogen add-back appears to be effective and safe in terms of pain relief and bone density[21].

In a 6-month placebo-controlled trial of goserelin and add-back hormone therapy, bone density loss was attenuated both during and after the completion of treatment in women treated with add-back therapy[22]. The mean percentage loss of bone mineral density at 6 months was 4.1% in controls, and 1.9 and 1.6% in the hormone replacement therapy (HRT) groups (0.3 mg conjugated oestrogen plus 5 mg medroxyprogesterone acetate and 0.625 mg conjugated oestrogen plus 5 mg medroxyprogesterone acetate). Bleeding patterns were similar in women in both groups and well tolerated, with only 11.3% drop-out over 6 months.

A large randomised placebo study examined the effects of three types of add-back treatment: norethindrone 5 mg daily, norethindrone plus premarin 0.625 mg daily, norethindrone plus premarin 1.25 mg daily, compared to placebo in 201 women administered depot leuprolide for 1 year[23]. All women had significant improvements in pelvic pain, although pain recurrence was highest in women on the higher 1.25-mg daily dose of premarin. Vasomotor symptoms were marked in the placebo group, and bone loss was measured as 3% at 6 months and 6% at 12 months. For the add-back therapy groups there was no significant bone loss, and the gonadotropin releasing hormone agonist adverse effects on lipid changes were corrected by the three types of add-back therapy.

A recently published review of the medical management of endometriosis-associated pain concluded that the oestrogen and progestogen components of add-back therapy should be as low as possible to reduce the risk of endometriosis recurrence and limit the negative effect on lipids. It also concluded that supplemental calcium should be administered at the same time[24]. The authors' recommendation is continuous combined low-dose hormone replacement therapy such as Livial® (tibolone) or Premique® (premarin 0.625 mg and medroxyprogesterone acetate 2 mg), which ensures amenorrhoea. This should be started during the mid-luteal phase of the menstrual cycle to reduce the flare effect and prevent an exacerbation of endometriosis-associated pain[25].

FUTURE MEDICAL TREATMENTS

Selective progesterone receptor modulators and progesterone antagonists

Many progesterone antagonists and selective progesterone receptor modulators display antiproliferative effects in the endometrium, which seem to be product- and dose-dependent. This property justifies their use in the treatment of fibroids and endometriosis. Selective progesterone receptor modulators such as asoprisnil are not as effective in blocking the luteinising hormone (LH) surge, and appear to target the endometrium directly and produce amenorrhoea. Treatment with these compounds is not associated with hypo-oestrogenism and bone loss.

Mifepristone

Mifepristone (RU486) is a progesterone antagonist which can inhibit ovulation and cause amenorrhoea. It is predominantly used in the medical management of miscarriage, although can reduce pelvic pain associated with endometriosis.

Aromatase inhibitors

Aromatase overexpression has recently been detected in endometriotic tissue. Aromatase (p450 arom) is responsible for converting C19 androgens into oestrogen in several types of human tissue. Aromatase activity causes local oestrogen biosynthesis, which in turn stimulates prostaglandin E_2 production by upregulating cyclo-oxygenase 2 (COX-2). Thus, a positive feedback cycle develops. In several human cell lines, prostaglandin and oestrogen concentrations are associated with proliferation, migration, angiogenesis, apoptosis resistance and even invasiveness. Consequently, aromatase and COX-2 are thought to be promising new treatments.

The aromatase inhibitor anastrazole, 1 mg daily combined with 20 μg of ethinyl oestradiol and 0.1 mg of levonorgestrel daily for 6 months, resulted in significant pain reduction in 14 of 15 women with refractory endometriosis-associated pain. Side-effects were mild and improved over time[26].

In a small non-randomised pilot study, vaginal anastrazole (0.25 mg daily for 6 months) was used for the treatment of histologically proven rectovaginal endometriosis. In a series of 10 women, dysmenorrhoea and physical and social functioning, but not chronic pelvic pain and dyspareunia, improved during treatment[27].

Gonadotropin releasing hormone antagonists

Gonadotropin releasing hormone antagonists have recently gained prominence in assisted conception cycles such as in vitro fertilisation (IVF). They result in immediate pituitary downregulation without the flare effect and potential reactivation of endometriosis. There are no long-acting preparations available, and they have not been subject to any comparative trials.

REFERENCES

1. Dawood MY. Dysmenorrhoea. J Reprod Med 1985; 30: 154–67.

2. Allen C, Hopewell S, Prentice A, Allen C. Non steroidal anti-inflammatory drugs for pain in women with endometriosis. Cochrane Database Syst Rev 2005; (4): CD004753.

3. Morrison BW, Daniels SE, Kotey P et al. Rofecoxib, a specific cyclooxygenase-2 inhibitor, in primary dysmenorrhoea: a randomized controlled trial. Obstet Gynecol 1999; 94: 504–8.

4. Robinson JL. Dysmenorrhoea and the use of oral contraceptives in adolescent women attending a family planning clinic. Am J Obstet Gynecol 1992; 166: 578–83.

5. Vercellini P, Trespidi L, Colombo A et al. A gonadotropin releasing hormone agonist versus a low dose oral contraceptive for pelvic pain associated with endometriosis. Fertil Steril 1993; 60: 75–9.

6. Vercellini P, De Giorgi O, Mosconi P et al. Cyproterone acetate versus a continuous monophasic oral contraceptive in the treatment of recurrent pain after conservative surgery for symptomatic endometriosis. Fertil Steril 2002; 77: 52–61

7. Luciano AA, Turksoy RN, Carleo J. Evaluation of oral medroxyprogesterone acetate in the treatment of endometriosis. Obstet Gynecol 1988; 72: 323–7

8. Moghissi KS, Boyce CRK. Management of endometriosis with oral medroxyprogesterone acetate. Obstet Gynecol 1976; 47: 265–7.

9. Roland M, Leisten D, Kane R. Endometriosis therapy with medroxyprogesterone acetate. J Reprod Med 1976; 17: 249–52.

10. Telimaa S, Puolakka J, Ronnberg L et al. Placebo-controlled comparison of danazol and high dose medroxyprogesterone acetate in the treatment of endometriosis. Gynecol Endocrinol 1987; 1: 13–23

11. Crosignani PG, Luciano A, Ray A, Bergqvist A. Subcutaneous medroxyprogesterone acetate versus leuprolide acetate in the treatment of endometriosis-associated pain. Hum Reprod 2006; 21: 248–56

12. Vercellini P, De Giogio O, Oldani S et al. Depot medroxyprogesterone acetate versus an oral contraceptive combined with very low dose danazol for long term treatment of pelvic pain associated with endometriosis. Am J Obstet Gynecol 1996; 175: 396–401.

13. Fedele L, Bianchi S, Zancanato G et al. Use of a levonorgestrel-releasing intrauterine device in the treatment of rectovaginal endometriosis. Fertil Steril 2001; 75: 485–8

14. Vercellini P, Aimi G, Panazza S et al. A levonorgestrel-releasing intrauterine system for the treatment of dysmenorrhea associated with endometriosis: a pilot study. Fertil Steril 1999; 72: 505–8

15. Petta CA, Ferriani RA, Abra MS et al. Randomized clinical trial of a levonorgestrel-releasing intrauterine system and a depot GnRH analogue for the treatment of chronic pelvic pain in women with endometriosis. Hum Reprod 2005; 20: 1993–8.

16. Dlugi AM, Miller JD, Knittle J. Lupron depot (leuprorelide acetate for depot suspension) in the treatment of endometriosis: a randomized placebo-controlled, double-blind study. Lupron study group. Fertil Steril 1990; 54: 419–27.

17. Bergqvist A, Bergh T, Hogström L et al. Effects of triptorelin versus placebo on the symptoms of endometriosis. Fertil Steril 1998; 69: 702–8.

18. Henzl MR, Corson SL, Moghissi K et al. Administration of nasal nafarelin as compared with oral danazol for endometriosis. A multicenter double-blind comparative clinical trial. N Engl J Med 1988; 318: 485–9.

19. Kennedy S, Barlow DH; Nafarelin European Endometriosis Trial Group (NEET). Nafarelin for endometriosis: a large-scale, danazol-controlled trial of efficacy and safety with 1-year follow-up. Fertil Steril 1992; 57: 514–22.

20. Ling F. Randomised controlled trial of depot leuprolide in patients with chronic pelvic pain and clinically suspected endometriosis. Pelvic Pain Study Group. Obstet Gynecol 1999; 93: 51–8.

21. Sagsveen M, Farmer JE, Prentice A, Breeze A. Gonadotrophin-releasing hormone analogues for endometriosis: bone mineral density. Cochrane Database Syst Rev 2003; (4): CD001297.

22. Moghissi KS, Schlaff WD, Olive DL, Skinner MA, Yin H. Goserelin acetate (Zoladex) with or without hormone replacement therapy for the treatment of endometriosis. Fertil Steril 1998; 69: 1056–62.

23. Hornstein MD, Surrey ES, Weisberg GW, Casino LA. Leuprolide acetate depot hormonal add-back in endometriosis: a 12-month study. Lupron Add-Back Study Group. Obstet Gynecol 1998; 91: 16–24.

24. Mahutte NG, Arici A. Medical management of endometriosis-associated pain. Obstet Gynecol Clin North Am 2003; 30:133–50.

25. Schattman GL. Treatment of chronic pelvic pain in patients with endometriosis [Comment]. Hum Reprod 2002; 17: 1128–9.

26. Amsterdam LL, Gentry W, Jobanputra S et al. Anastrazole and oral contraceptives: a novel treatment for endometriosis. Fertil Steril 2005; 84: 300–4.

27. Hefler LA, Grimm C, Trotsenburg M, Nagele F. Role of the vaginally administered aromatase inhibitor anastrazole in women with rectovaginal endometriosis: a pilot study. Fertil Steril 2005; 84: 1033–6.

CHAPTER 9

Surgical treatment of endometriosis

IMPORTANCE OF ADEQUATE LAPAROSCOPIC EXAMINATION

It is apparent that endometriosis has a wide variety of visual appearances and only careful laparoscopic assessment of the pelvis will reveal these features.

In the majority of instances, the laparoscopic appearances of endometriotic implants are characteristic and diagnosis is simple, without the need for biopsy. Biopsy may be necessary with the non-pigmented and opacified implants to confirm the diagnosis. The surgeon should look for bluish-black implants or papules varying in colour on or under the peritoneal surface, and for deep infiltrating implants in the pouch of Douglas, on and around the uterosacral ligaments and posterior wall of the uterus, under the ovary in the ovarian fossae and rectovaginal septum (Figures 9.1 and 9.2).

Inspection of the pelvis should be carried out in a logical and systematic way (Figures 9.3–9.17). A second port and instrument are needed to lift the ovaries and fully inspect the pelvis. First, the liver and diaphragms are inspected to look for perihepatic adhesions, which suggest infective rather than endometriotic pathology. Inspect the uterovesical fold and lift the uterus forward into anteversion. Move the bowel out of the pouch of Douglas. Fluid in the pouch should be aspirated to ensure that implants are not missed. Inspect both tubes and ovaries. Using an instrument through the second port, lift the ovaries to ensure that they are mobile and inspect the undersurface and peritoneum of the ovarian fossae. Examine both uterosacral ligaments, the pouch of Douglas and the back of the uterus. Deep, infiltrating endometriotic implants are often better palpated than visualised. This can be done with a blunt probe or graspers through the second port. In the authors' opinion, use of the Veress needle as a second instrument is inadequate for this reason. With advanced endometriosis and massive adhesion formation between the reproductive and neighbouring organs, it may become difficult or impossible to identify endometriotic implants. However, it is usually possible to identify typical implants in some area within the pelvis to enable confirmation of the disease.

SURGICAL MANAGEMENT OF ENDOMETRIOSIS

Laparoscopy allows a diagnosis of endometriosis to be made along with an assessment of the extent of disease. With the advent of improved laparoscopic equipment and enhanced surgical techniques, complex conservative surgery can now be performed safely. In severe cases where bowel, bladder and ureter are involved, laparotomy may be required, and sometimes the assistance of surgical colleagues. The aim of surgery is to remove or destroy visible and/or palpable endometriosis with the specific aim of improving pelvic pain and enhancing fertility.

The extent of surgery is dependent on the preoperative symptoms, the severity of disease, the wishes of the patient and the need for informed consent. Most clinicians use the revised American Fertility Society (AFS) scoring system for endometriosis, comprising four groups: minimal (stage I), mild (stage II), moderate (stage III) and severe (stage IV), according to the operative findings[1]. Various treatment modalities are available for use at laparoscopic surgery. These include: laser, scissors with monopolar electrocautery and bipolar coagulation, harmonic scalpel. All allow resection, cauterisation and vaporisation of endometriosis.

The failure rate of surgery alone, in terms of pain relief, is significant. Results have consistently shown that 30–40% of women will not have any improvement or will have recurrence despite surgery. Improvement rates published in the literature vary from 44 to 81%, which changes according to the length of follow-up. In a study by Keye and colleagues[2], there was an initial improvement of 92%, but 32% had recurrence at 9 months.

Sutton and co-workers[3] conducted a randomised, double-blind trial of laser ablation for endometriosis-associated pelvic pain. Six months after surgery, 63% of those treated with laser ablation and/or laparoscopic uterosacral nerve ablation (LUNA) had an improvement in their pain compared to 23% who had diagnostic laparoscopy only. In other words, 37% of women had no benefit from surgery in terms of reduction in pain. For minimal disease, only 38%

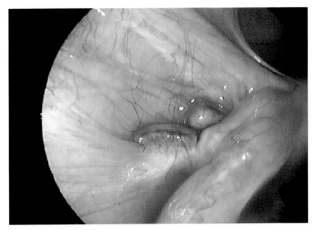

Figure 9.1 Blue-black endometriotic deposit

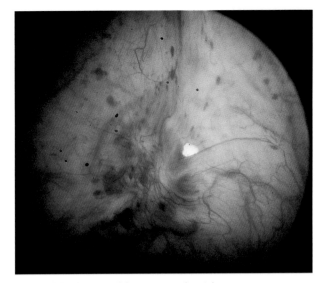

Figure 9.2 New vessel formation and vesicles

(a)

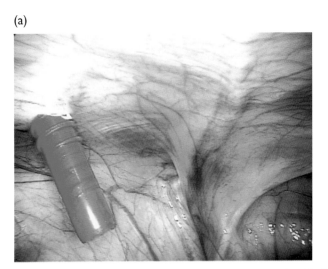

(b)

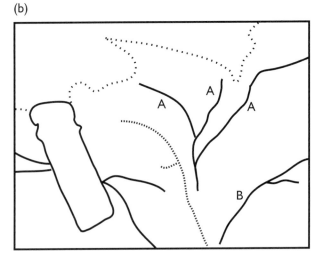

Figure 9.3 (a, b) A second port and instrument are needed to lift the ovaries and fully inspect the pelvis. The epigastric vessels (A) can be located lateral to the obliterated umbilical artery (B)

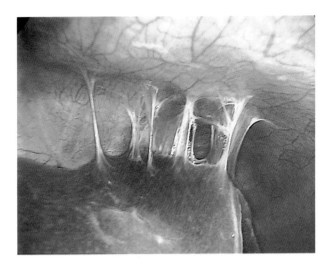

Figure 9.4 Inspection of the liver and diaphragms. Perihepatic adhesions suggest infective aetiology

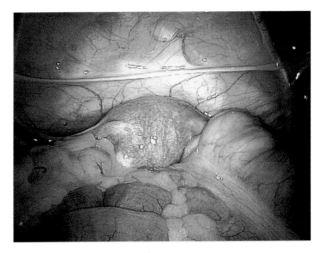

Figure 9.5 Uterus in retroversion

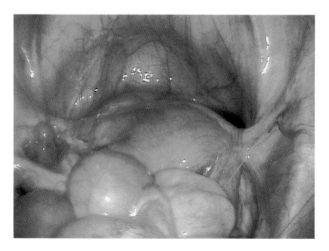

Figure 9.6 The uterovesical fold before anteversion fails to detect the severe endometriosis and obliteration of the pouch of Douglas

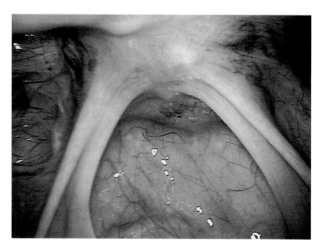

Figure 9.9 Close-up view of the uterosacral ligaments

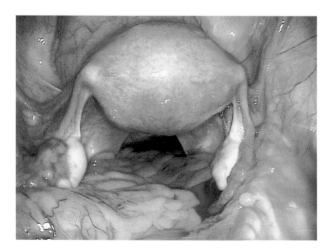

Figure 9.7 Uterus in anteversion giving panoramic view of the pelvis

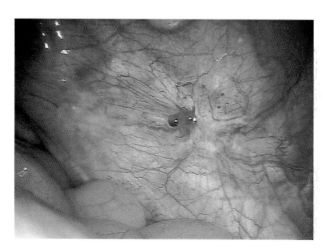

Figure 9.10 It is important to aspirate any fluid in order to fully inspect the pouch of Douglas

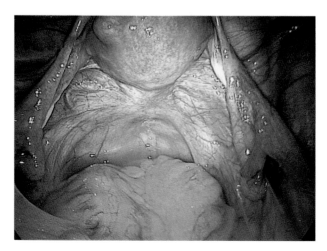

Figure 9.8 Uterus in anteversion

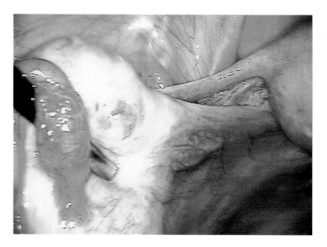

Figure 9.11 The left ovary is lifted with a second instrument to inspect the ovarian fossa

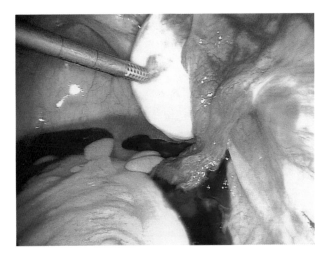

Figure 9.12 Normal patent right fallopian tube

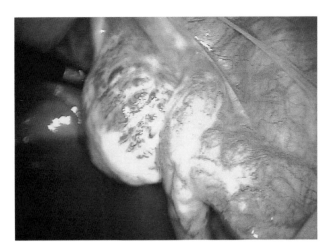

Figure 9.15 Superficial ovarian endometriosis. It is necessary to lift up the ovary to ensure that it is mobile and inspect the under-surface and peritoneum in the ovarian fossa

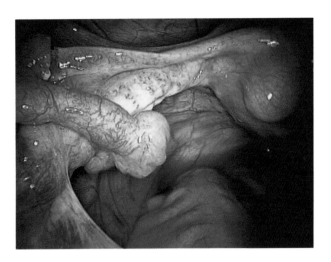

Figure 9.13 Normal left tube and ovary

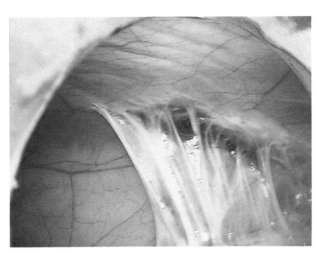

Figure 9.16 Adhesions to the undersurface of the Pfannenstiel scar secondary to endometriosis

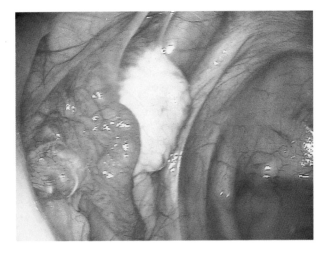

Figure 9.14 The left ovary and ovarian fossa with the left ureter visible

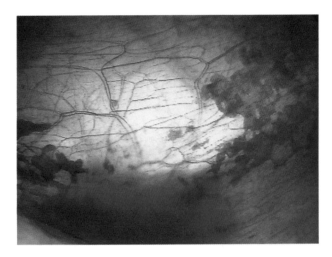

Figure 9.17 Haemosiderin staining of the uterovesical peritonem

of women had a reduction in pain. Thus, surgery is more effective in reducing pain in women with more severe disease.

Sutton and colleagues published the results of the longer follow-up in 1997[4]. One year after the initial surgery, 44%, almost half of the treated women, had recurrence of pain requiring additional treatment. Surgical failure may result from missed lesions, incomplete resection, recurrence of disease or the pain due to an alternative aetiology. Surgery must be considered cytoreductive, and although there is no randomised trial, as much deep disease as possible must be removed to achieve the best possible outcome.

PREOPERATIVE ASSESSMENT

Careful preoperative assessment enables a clinical staging and possible surgical difficulties to be anticipated. This is essential in giving informed consent, particularly where fertility is desired and treatment must be conservative.

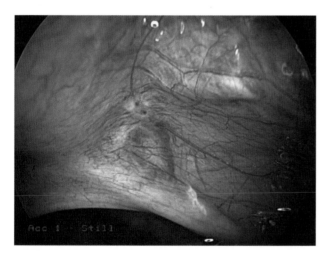

Figure 9.18 Active endometriotic deposit in the left ovarian fossa

It is essential that the woman understands what surgery will involve and has a realistic idea of what surgery can achieve.

If the uterus is mobile, a preoperative ultrasound scan to exclude an endometrioma may be sufficient preoperative investigation. CA 125 may assist in postoperative management, particularly if elevated preoperatively.

If there is nodularity and/or tenderness of the uterosacral ligaments or cul-de-sac, deeply infiltrating disease should be suspected. In addition to the investigations above, ultrasound of the kidneys and renal tract should be carried out. If dyschezia is a symptom, a barium enema and/or sigmoidoscopy to assess bowel involvement should be considered.

Bowel preparation should be undertaken where clinical findings and imaging reveal that advanced disease with bowel involvement is present. It may also be appropriate to carry out surgery with a multidisciplinary team involving the gynaecologists and the colorectal surgeons.

Venous thromboembolic prophylaxis should be given, as well as antibiotic prophylaxis. Bacteraemia is not uncommon after prolonged pelvic surgery, and antibiotic cover is advisable.

Minimal and mild endometriosis

These two groups of endometriosis more often involve the superficial peritoneal covering of the pelvic organs (Figures 9.18–9.23). They are usually treated with coagulation or laser vaporisation of the endometriotic implants.

A randomised trial attempted to answer the question as to whether endometriosis should be excised or ablated[5]. Both produced good symptom relief and a reduction in pelvic tenderness. There was no difference in morbidity; one woman from each group became pregnant during the study period. Two participants reported no relief or a worsening of symptoms or signs.

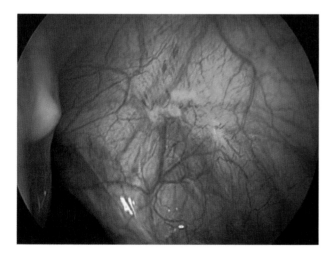

Figure 9.19 Prominent neovascularisation

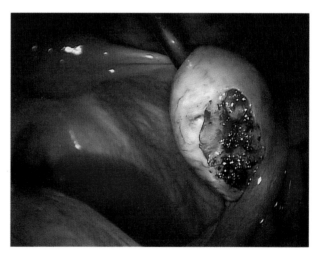

Figure 9.20 Diathermy of superficial endometriosis

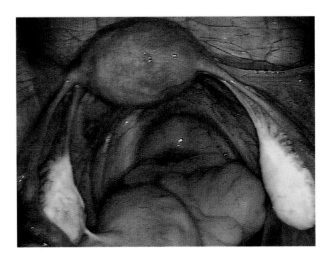

Figure 9.21 Bowel adherent to the left ovary secondary to superficial endometriosis

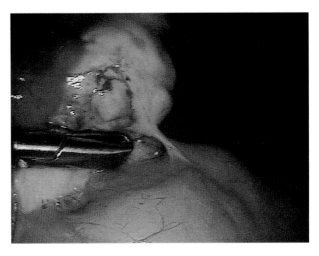

Figure 9.22 Close-up view of the same patient as in Figure 9.21

Moderate and severe endometriosis

These two groups relate to the extensive presence of endometriosis within the pelvis, but this does not always correlate to the severity of pelvic pain, especially dysmenorrhoea[6]. Deep infiltrating endometriosis is present when endometriosis penetrates greater than 5 mm under the peritoneal surface[7]. It can involve the uterosacral ligaments, the posterior vaginal wall and anterior rectal wall[8]. The presence of deep infiltrating endometriosis requires careful pelvic examination to identify the lesions, and does not always correlate with a high revised AFS score. A recent study demonstrated that the severity of pelvic pain, in particular dysmenorrhoea, correlated to the depth of involvement of deep infiltrating endometriosis[9]. The frequency and severity of deep dyspareunia correlates to uterosacral involvement, whereas non-cyclical chronic pelvic pain is more common when there is bowel involvement[10]. To reduce pelvic pain and prevent recurrence of symptoms, surgery would require excision of the endometriotic lesions as well as coagulation or laser vaporisation of more superficial endometriotic implants.

Deep fibrotic endometriosis involving the pouch of Douglas requires an excision of the nodular fibrotic deposit(s) from the posterior vagina, rectum, posterior cervix and uterosacral ligaments. Complete dissection of the anterior rectum is required until the loose connective tissue of the rectovaginal space is reached. A sponge on a forceps is inserted into the posterior fornix and a dilator (size 25) inserted into the rectum to delineate the structures. In addition, a cannula is inserted into the endometrial cavity to antevert the uterus. The peritoneum covering the pouch of Douglas is opened between the nodule and the rectum and excision of the fibrotic nodule on the side of the rectum attempted only after rectal dissection is complete. In deeply infiltrating lesions, the vaginal wall is more or less penetrated by the endometriosis, and excision of a part of the vagina is essential (Figures 9.24–9.41).

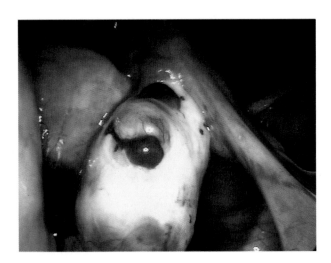

Figure 9.23 Right ovarian endometrioma

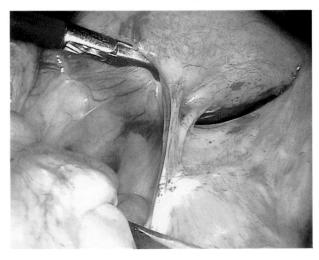

Figure 9.24 Bowel adhesion to the posterior surface of the uterus

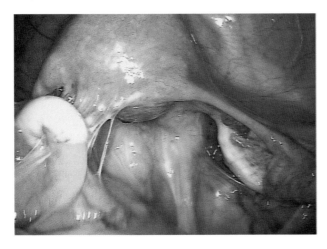

Figure 9.25 Bowel adhesions to the left adnexa and obliterated pouch of Douglas. It is possible to feel a nodule vaginally

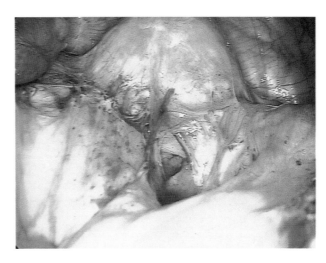

Figure 9.28 Extensive bowel adhesions and obliteration of the pouch of Douglas

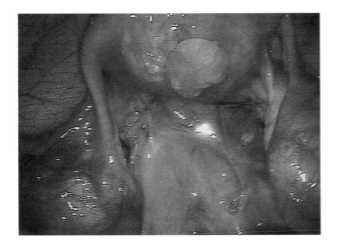

Figure 9.26 Obliterated pouch of Douglas

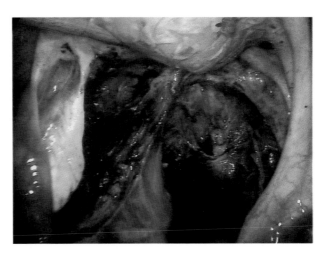

Figure 9.29 Exensive excision of deep rectovaginal endometriosis and uterosacral ligaments. The left ureter can be seen

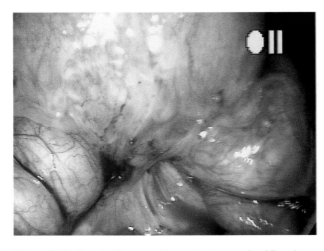

Figure 9.27 Bowel adhesions obliterating the pouch of Douglas

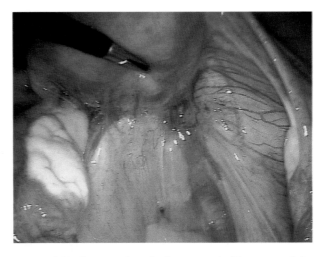

Figure 9.30 Extensive bowel adhesions and obliteration of the pouch of Douglas

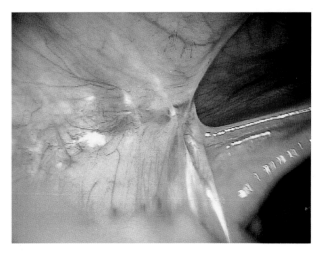

Figure 9.31 Bowel adhesion obscuring the left adnexa

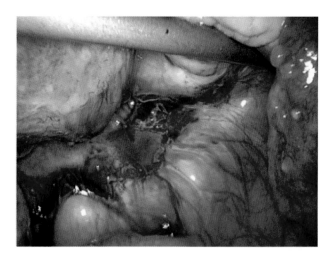

Figure 9.34 Initial disssection confirms deep infiltrating endometriosis

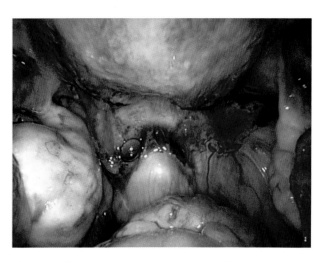

Figure 9.32 Extensive active endometriosis with partial obliteration of the pouch of Douglas

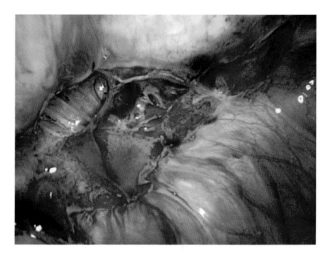

Figure 9.35 Continuing dissection

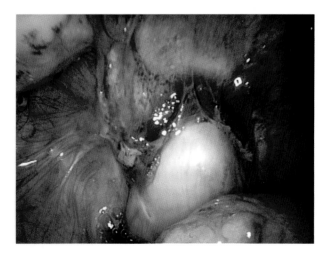

Figure 9.33 Close-up of view shown in Figure 9.32

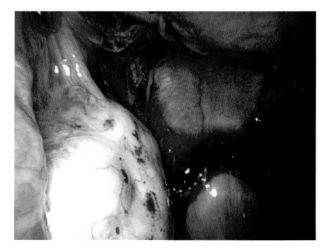

Figure 9.36 Mobilisation of the left ovary

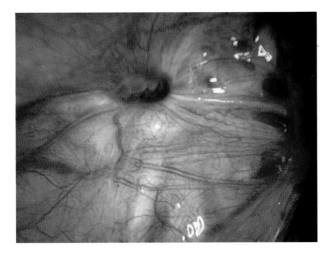

Figure 9.37 Peritoneal side wall below the left ovary

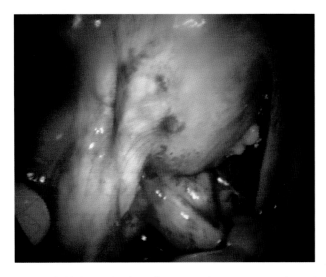

Figure 9.40 Sigmoid colon adherent to the posterior surface of the uterus

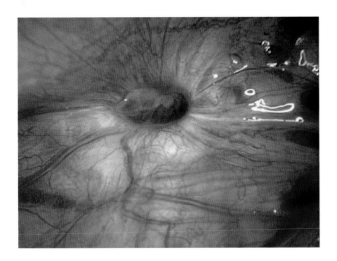

Figure 9.38 Close-up of view shown in Figure 9.37

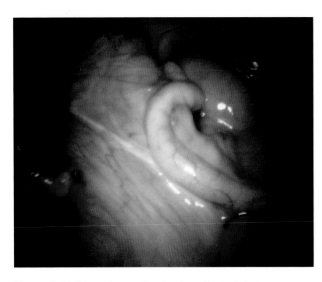

Figure 9.41 Normal appendix after bowel adhesiolysis

Endometrioma management

Endometriomas are endometriotic ovarian cysts, and often associated with moderate to severe endometriosis. Their management is controversial. The objectives are to reduce pelvic pain, prevent recurrence and enhance fertility. Small endometriomas, less than 5 mm, are normally drained and coagulated, but can be vaporised or excised[11]. In a randomised controlled trial, laparoscopic cystectomy was shown to significantly reduce pelvic pain and prevent recurrence compared to laparoscopic drainage alone[12]. An alternative method is to perform laparoscopic cyst fenestration and ablation of the cyst capsule. Any coexisting endometriosis should also be treated. This has been shown to significantly improve pelvic pain, with a very high patient satisfaction rating[13] (Figures 9.42–9.45).

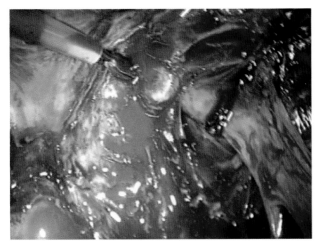

Figure 9.39 Dissection of the right ureter

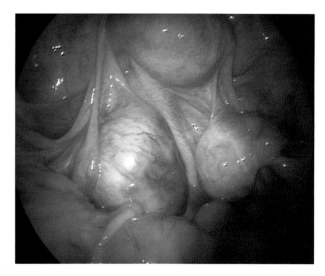

Figure 9.42 Large left endometrioma

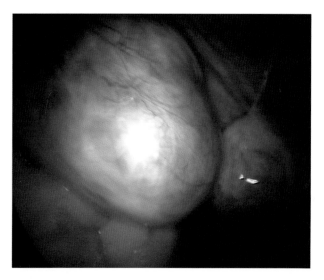

Figure 9.43 Close-up of the left ovarian endometrioma from Figure 9.42

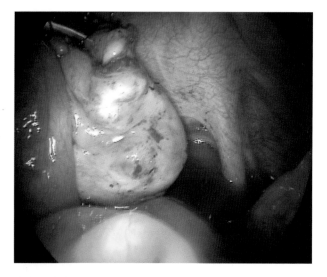

Figure 9.44 The reconstructed left ovary after formal laparoscopic ovarian cystectomy

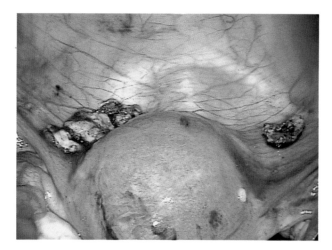

Figure 9.45 The uterovesical fold is convenient to keep any surgical specimen

Laparoscopic uterine nerve ablation

Medical treatment for dysmenorrhoea includes the oral contraceptive pill, non-steroidal anti-inflammatory drugs and the levonorgestrel-releasing intrauterine system. While these treatments are successful, there is still a 20–25% failure rate, and surgery is an option for such women. Five trials investigated laparoscopic uterine nerve ablation (LUNA) with some evidence of effectiveness when compared to control or no treatment. The treatment of laparoscopic uterine nerve ablation combined with surgical treatment of endometrial implants versus surgical treatment of endometriosis alone did not aid pain relief[14].

LUNA involves transection of both uterosacral ligaments with the specific aim of disrupting the efferent nerve fibres supplying the uterus. The technique remains controversial, as there is no good evidence to demonstrate that it is effective. In a double-blind randomised controlled study, the addition of LUNA to laparoscopic laser vaporisation of endometriosis was not found to improve pelvic pain[15]. The authors believe that this procedure should not be performed if the uterosacral ligaments have a normal appearance. In the presence of deep infiltrating endometriotic lesions on the uterosacral ligaments, excision is advised (Figures 9.46–9.52).

Laparoscopic presacral neurectomy

This technique aims to disrupt the hypogastric plexus and relieve chronic pelvic pain. In selected cases it has been shown to be effective at treating dysmenorrhoea and chronic pelvic pain[16]. A recent prospective observational study of 15 patients with minimal to moderate endometriosis demonstrated that laparoscopic presacral chemical neurolysis with phenol resulted in a reduction of total pelvic pain, especially dysmenorrhoea, and an improvement in sexual function[17]. It appeared to be a safe procedure, with the most common side-effect being constipation.

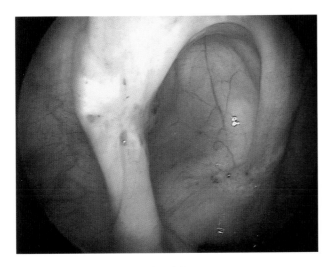

Figurer 9.46 Left uterosacral nodule

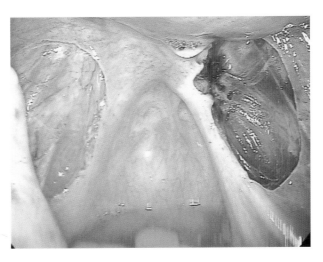

Figure 9.49 Excision of the uterosacral ligaments and bilateral uterosacral nodules

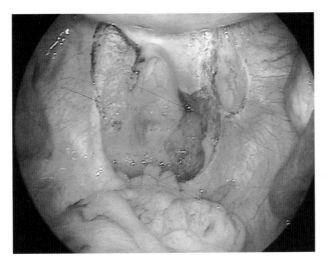

Figure 9.47 After excision of the nodule in the same patient as in Figure 9.46

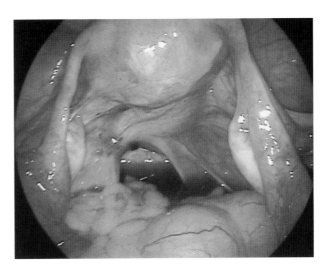

Figure 9.50 Nodule in the pouch of Douglas with tethering of bowel

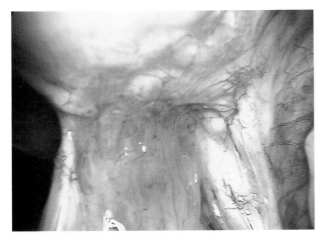

Figure 9.48 Obliterated pouch of Douglas. Deep nodule involving the left uterosacral ligament

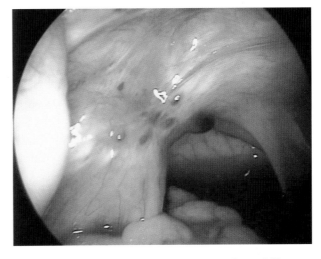

Figure 9.51 Close-up of the same patient as in Figure 9.50

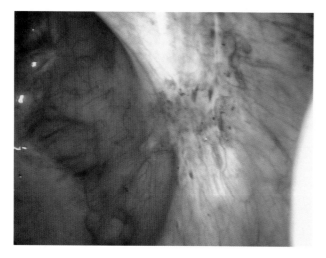

Figure 9.52 Right uterosacral nodule

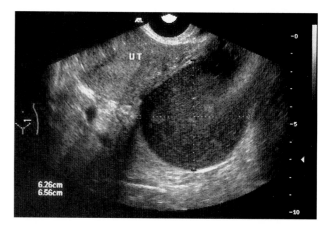

Figure 9.53 Ultrasound image of left ovarian endometrioma

A trial of presacral neurectomy combined with endometriosis treatment versus endometriosis treatment alone showed that there was an overall improvement in pain relief. The data suggest that this may be specific for midline abdominal pain only. Adverse events were significantly more common for presacral neurectomy, but the majority were constipation, which may improve spontaneously[14].

Laparotomy, hysterectomy with or without oophorectomy

In some cases of severe endometriosis laparoscopic surgery is not possible and laparotomy is required to tackle extensive adhesions especially involving the bowel, bladder and ureter. For women who have completed their families and who have severe pain despite other treatments, hysterectomy is an option. It is the complete excision of deeply infiltrating endometriosis that is key to the reduction of pain[18].

Oophorectomy should only be considered once it is clear that the ovaries are contributing to the pelvic pain (Figures 9.53–9.55). It is sometimes helpful to administer a 3-month course of gonadotropin releasing hormone agonists to induce amenorrhoea and a short-term cessation of ovarian function. The resolution of pain suggests that oophorectomy will provide long-term pain relief. Continuation of the pain suggests that the pain is due to other causes.

Hormone replacement therapy (HRT) is recommended after bilateral oophorectomy in young women, given the overall health benefits and small risk of recurrent disease while taking HRT. The ideal regimen is unclear. Adding a progestogen after hysterectomy is unnecessary, but may protect against the unopposed action of oestrogen on any residual disease. The theoretical benefit of avoiding disease reactivation or malignant transformation should be balanced against the increase in breast cancer reported to be associated with combined oestrogen and progestogen HRT and tibolone.

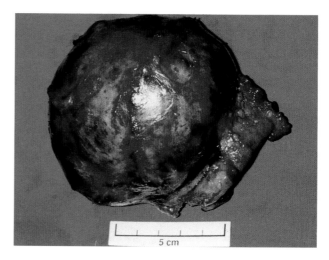

Figure 9.54 Left ovarian endometrioma after surgical excision

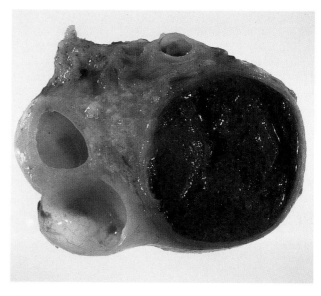

Figure 9.55 A chocolate cyst in an ovary containing other smaller fibrous-lined cyst cavities

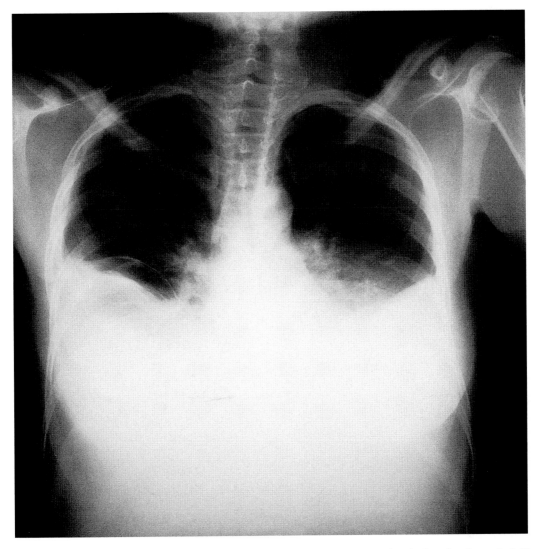

Figure 9.56 Bilateral haemothoraces. These coincided with menstruation and were associated with pleural endometriosis. The patient presented with cyclical chest pain

COMBINED MEDICAL AND SURGICAL MANAGEMENT

Unless medical treatment is being given as an adjunct to surgical treatment, laparoscopy should not be carried out during or within 3 months of medical treatment so as to avoid underdiagnosis.

There are some retrospective data demonstrating benefit of medical treatment prior to surgery for moderate to severe endometriosis[19]. There are, however, good data confirming that postoperative medical treatment with gonadotropin releasing hormone agonists for 6 months significantly reduces pelvic pain and delays recurrence by more than 12 months[20,21]. A recent consensus statement from an expert panel concluded that the balance of evidence supports the use of adjuvant postoperative medical therapy after conservative surgery for chronic pelvic pain due to moderate to severe endometriosis[22].

RECURRENT ENDOMETRIOSIS

In a two year follow up study of 311 women with newly diagnosed endometriosis, the recurrence rate of clinically detectable endometriosis tended to be higher in older women with advanced stages of the disease and lower in women with infertility. The 2-year recurrence rate was 5.7% among cases I–II and 14.4% among stage III–IV. The recurrence rates tended to increase with age, being 4.6% among women aged 20–30 and 13.1% among women aged over 30 years[23].

Trends in hospital utilisation and surgical rates for endometriosis and readmission over 4 years among women with minimal–mild endometriosis suggested that 27% of women required readmission within 4 years for additional surgical treatment, and the risk of having a hysterectomy was 12%[24].

Treatment of recurrent endometriosis depends on the symptoms, fertility wishes and previous treatment. Women

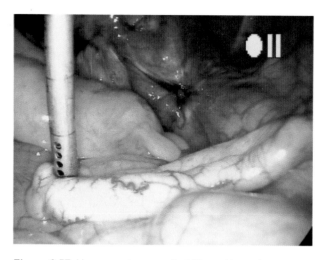

Figure 9.57 Hypervascular appendix infiltrated by endometriosis

treated medically should be offered repeat laparoscopy with the option of surgical treatment. Where there are endometriomas and deeply infiltrating endometriosis, it may be practical to carry out ovarian cystectomy followed by excision of deeply infiltrating disease in the cul-de-sac. This approach would allow both assessment and treatment and the opportunity for informed consent. When there are severe symptoms and repeated recurrence, a radical surgical approach may be the best option for long-term pain relief.

EXTRAPELVIC ENDOMETRIOSIS

Extrapelvic endometriosis is rare, and can affect many sites (Figures 9.56–9.79).

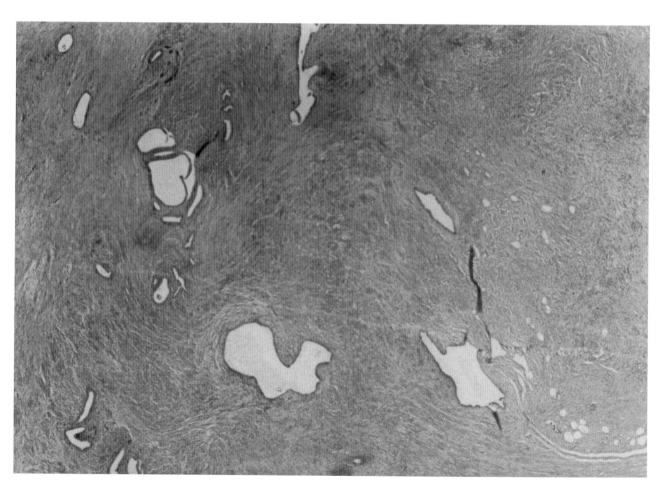

Figure 9.58 Appendiceal lumen obliterated by endometriosis

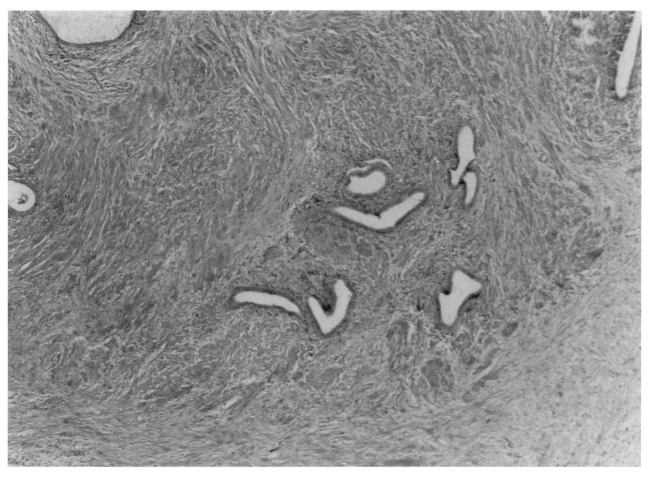

Figure 9.59 Appendiceal muscularis infiltrated by endometriosis

MALIGNANT CHANGE WITHIN ENDOMETRIOSIS

Malignant change within endometriosis is rare, but well documented (Figure 9.80).

EXPECTANT MANAGEMENT OF ENDOMETRIOSIS

The natural history of endometriosis is uncertain, as the disease may improve as well as deteriorate without treatment[25]. Expectant management may be reasonable if the finding of endometriosis is incidental and the woman is in her 40s and has completed her family. A long-term study of women identified with endometriosis at the time of laparoscopic sterilisation found that pelvic pain did not become a problem, compared to endometriosis-free controls[26]. The prevalence of endometriosis in this group of women was 20%, with the majority having mild endometriosis according to the revised AFS score.

CONCLUSIONS

The management of endometriosis-associated pain is dependent on the severity of symptoms, the stage of endometriosis, family plans and informed consent. Medical treatments mainly rely on hormonal manipulation of the ovarian cycle and exert their effect by inducing amenorrhoea. They are all effective in reducing endometriosis-associated pain, but are contraceptive and can have significant side-effects which preclude long-term use. The oral contraceptive pill, Mirena® intrauterine system or continuous progestins are generally used as first-line treatment. They are generally well tolerated and can be continued in the long term. If they are unsuccessful in alleviating pain and improving quality of life, second-line treatment would be gonadotropin releasing hormone agonists with add-back continuous combined hormone replacement therapy.

Conservative laparoscopic surgery is effective in reducing endometriosis-associated pelvic pain as well as enhancing

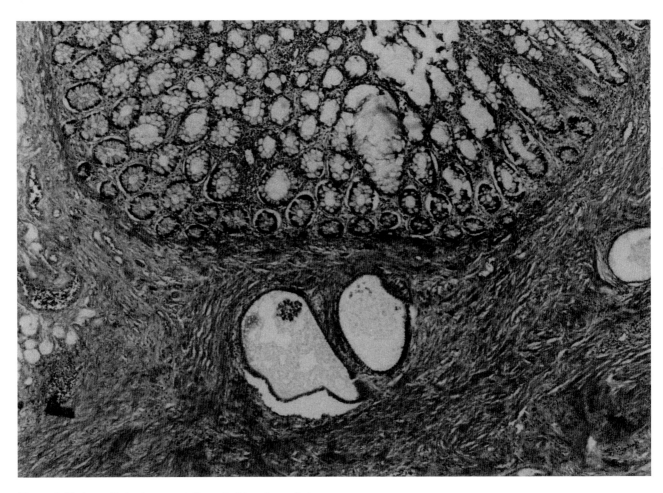

Figure 9.60 Appendical submucosa infiltrated with endometriosis

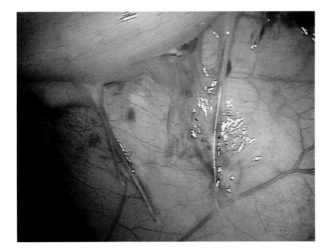

Figure 9.61 Vesicular implants on small bowel

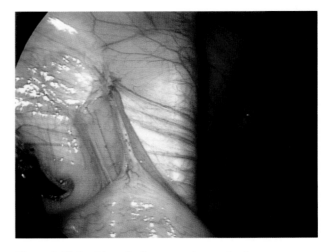

Figure 9.62 Small bowel adherent to the ovarian fossa

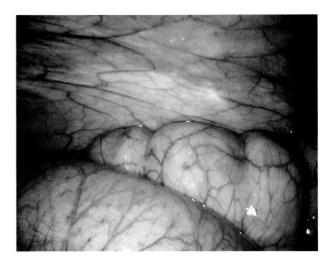

Figure 9.63 Hypervascularisation of the bowel

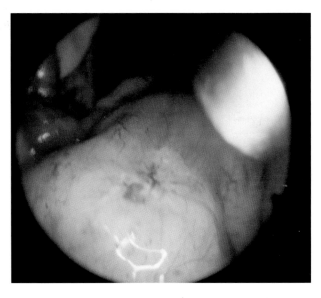

Figure 9.64 Superficial, vascular active endometriotic deposit on the serosal surface of the sigmoid. One lesion has been vaporised with CO_2 ultrapulse laser. (Courtesy of Professor C Sutton)

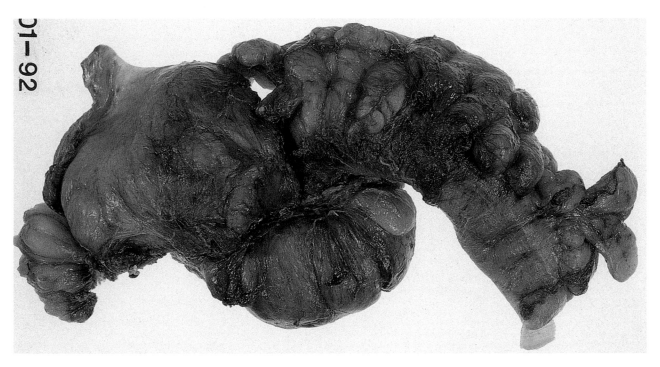

Figure 9.65 Endometriosis of the sigmoid colon. The patient (known to have endometriosis) presented with cyclical rectal bleeding, increasing dyschezia and tenesmus, and was admitted with obstruction of the large bowel

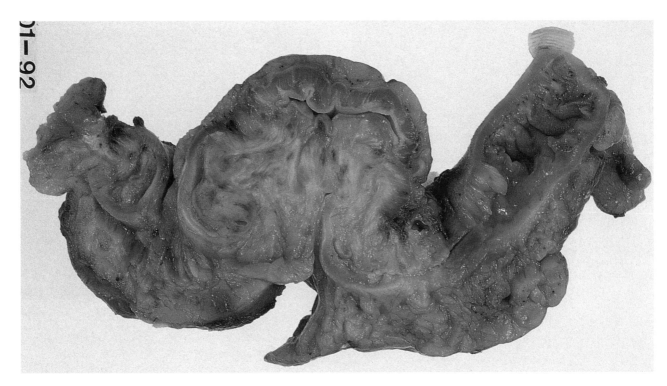

Figure 9.66 Stricture within the colon, increased fibrosis and polypoidal projection of the colon into the mesentery wall with areas of haemorrhage within the wall

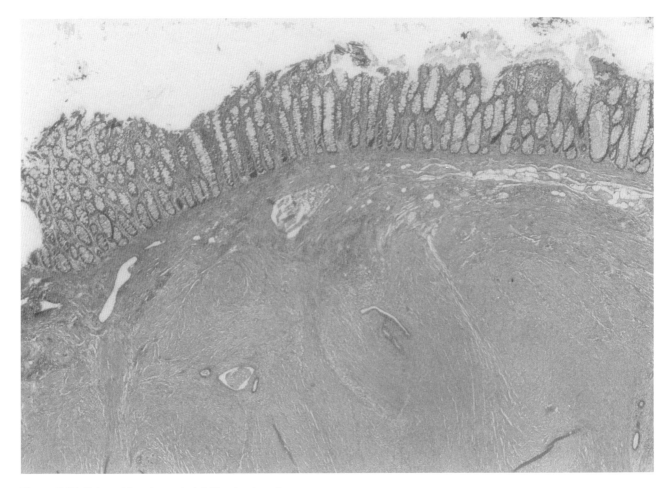

Figure 9.67 Colon with endometriosis infiltrating the submucosa

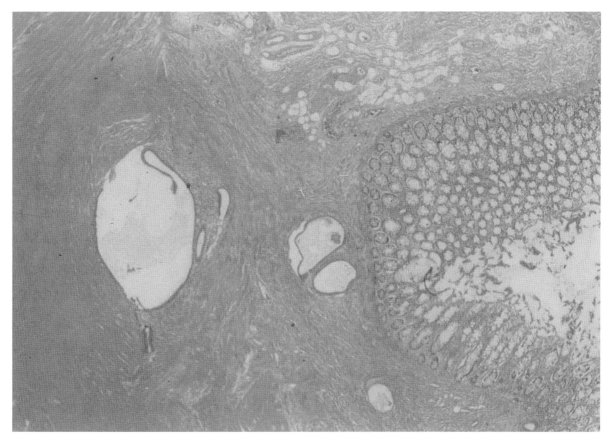

Figure 9.68 Endometriosis infiltrating a gland in the descending colon

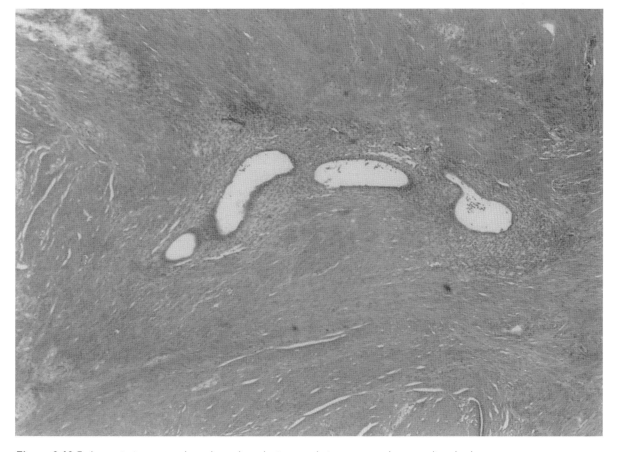

Figure 9.69 Endometriosis present throughout the colonic muscularis mucosa and surrounding glands

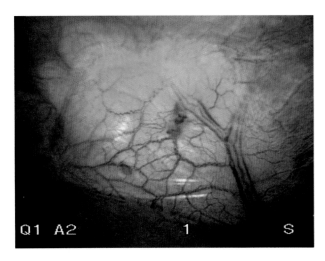

Figure 9.70 Endometriosis on the diaphragm with extensive neovascularisation

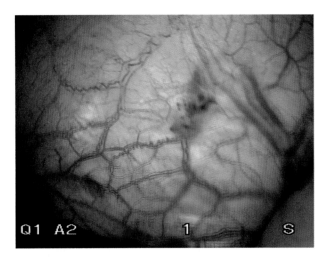

Figure 9.71 Higher magnification of Figure 9.70 showing diaphragmatic endometriosis with neovascularisation

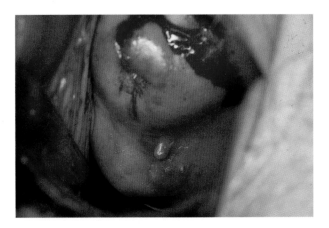

Figure 9.72 Endometriosis involving the posterior vaginal fornix. The deep endometriosis was continuous with lesions in the pouch of Douglas. (Courtesy of Mr Bromham)

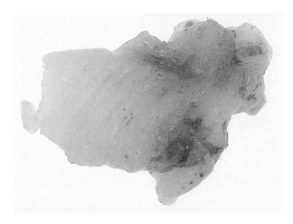

Figure 9.73 Excised vaginal vault endometriotic lesion

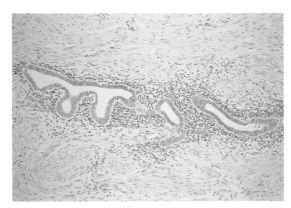

Figure 9.74 Histology from vaginal vault lesions, with endometriotic foci showing poor activity, (the patient had received gonadotropin releasing hormone analogues for 4 months preoperatively)

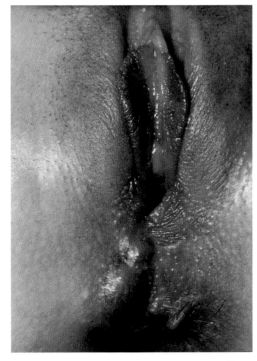

Figure 9.75 Endometriosis in an episiotomy scar. The patient presented with a cyclical, tender swelling in the perineum. (Courtesy of Mr D Bromham)

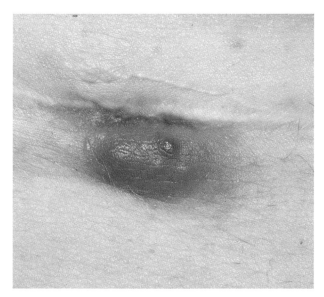

Figurre 9.76 Superfical endometriotic deposit in Caesarean section scar. The patient presented with a cyclical, painful nodule in the scar. (Courtesy of Mr D Bromham and Professor J Scott)

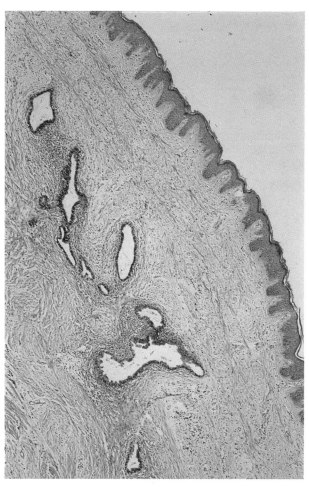

Figure 9.78 Histology of biopsy from endometriosis in the anterior abdominal wall showing glandular elements beneath the skin (H&E, X90)

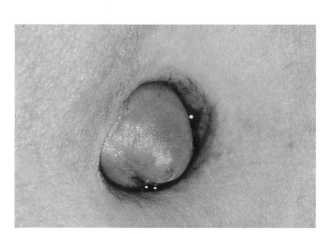

Figure 9.77 Endometriosis involving the umbilicus in a patient with extensive pelvic recurrent endometriosis. The patient presented with cyclical pain and bleeding from the umbilicus (Courtesy of Mr D Bromham)

fertility. The body of evidence currently favours a minimum of 6-month postoperative medical treatment for moderate to severe endometriosis, as this delays the recurrence of pelvic pain and improves the quality of life.

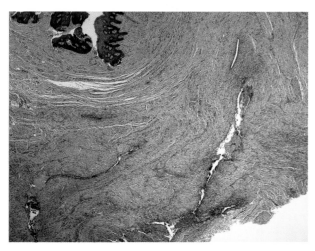

Figure 9.79 Endometriosis within an episiotomy scar

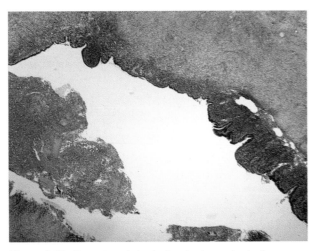

Figure 9.80 Clustering of glands showing hyperplastic changes

REFERENCES

1. The American Fertility Society. Revised American Fertility Society classification of endometriosis: 1985. Fertil Steril 1985; 43: 351–2.

2. Keye WR Jr, Hansen LW, Astin M, Poulson AM Jr. Argon laser therapy of endometriosis: a review of 92 consecutive patients. Fertil Steril 1987; 47: 208–12.

3. Sutton CJ, Ewen SP, Whitelaw N, Haines P. Prospective random-ized, double-blind controlled trial of laser laparoscopy in the treatment of pelvic pain associated with minimal, mild and mod-erate endometriosis. Fertil Steril 1994; 62: 696–700.

4. Sutton CJ, Polley AS, Ewen SP, Haines P. Follow-up report on a randomized, double-blind controlled trial of laser laparoscopy in the treatment of pelvic pain associated with minimal, mild and moderate endometriosis. Fertil Steril 1997; 68: 1070–4.

5. Wright J, Lotfallah H, Jones K, Lovell D. A randomized trial of excision versus ablation for mild endometriosis. Fertil Steril 2005; 83: 1830–6.

6. Porpora MG. Koninckx PR, Piazze J et al. Correlation between endometriosis and pelvic pain. J Am Assoc Gynecol Laparosc 1999; 6: 429–34.

7. Koninckx PR, Martin DC. Treatment of deeply infiltrating endometriosis. Curr Opin Obstet Gynecol 1994; 6: 231–41.

8. Chapron C, Fauconnier A, Vieira M et al. Anatomic distribution of deeply infiltrating endometriosis: surgical implications and proposition for a classification. Hum Reprod 2003; 18: 157–61.

9. Chapron C, Fauconnier A, Dubuisson J-B et al. Deep infiltrating endometriosis: relation between severity of dysmenorrhoea and extent of disease. Hum Reprod 2003; 18: 760–6.

10. Fauconnier A, Chapron C, Dubuisson J-B et al. Relation between pain symptoms and the anatomic location of deep infiltrating endometriosis. Fertil Steril 2002; 78: 719–26.

11. Martin DC, O'Conner DT. Surgical management of endometrio-sis-associated pain. Obstet Gynecol Clin North Am 2003; 30: 151–62.

12. Beretta P, Franchi M, Ghezzi F et al. Randomised clinical trial of two laparoscopic treatments of endometriomas: cystectomy versus drainage and coagulation. Fertil Steril 1998; 70: 1176–80.

13. Jones KD, Sutton C. Patient satisfaction and changes in pain scores after ablative laparoscopic surgery for stage III–IV endometriosis and endometriotic cysts. Fertil Steril 2003; 79: 1086–90.

14. Proctor M, Latthe P, Farquhar C, Khan K, Johnson N. Surgical interruption of pelvic nerve pathways for primary and secondary dysmenorrhoea. Cochrane Database Syst Rev 2005; (4): CD001896.

15. Sutton C, Pooley AS, Jones KD, et al. A prospective, randomised, double-blind controlled trial of laparoscopic uterine nerve abla-tion in the treatment of pelvic pain associated with endometrio-sis. Gynecol Endosc 2001; 10: 217–22.

16. Kwok A, Lam A, Ford R. Laparoscopic presacral neurectomy: a review. Obstet Gynecol Surv 2001; 56: 99–104.

17. Soysal ME, Soysal S, Gurses E, Ozer S. Laparoscopic presacral neurolysis for endometriosis-related pelvic pain. Hum Reprod 2003; 18: 588–92.

18. Chopin N, Viera M, Borghese B et al. Operative management of deeply infiltrating endometriosis: results on pelvic pain symp-toms according to a surgical classification. J Minim Invasive Gynecol 2005; 12: 106–12.

19. Donnez J, Lemaire-Rubbers M, Karaman Y et al. Combined (hormonal and microsurgical) therapy in infertile women with endometriosis. Fertil Steril 1987; 48: 239–42.

20. Vercellini P, Crosignani PG, Fadini R et al. A gonadotrophin-releasing hormone agonist compared with expectant manage-ment after conservative surgery for symptomatic endometriosis. Br J Obstet Gynaecol 1999; 106: 672–7.

21. Hornstein MD, Hemmings R, Yuzpe AA, Heinrichs WL. Use of naferelin versus placebo after reductive laparoscopic surgery for endometriosis. Fertil Steril 1997; 68: 860–4.

22. Gambone JC, Mittman BS, Munro MG et al. Consensus state-ment for the management of chronic pelvic pain and endometriosis: proceedings of an expert-panel consensus process. Fertil Steril 2002; 78: 961–72.

23. Parazzini F, Bertulessi C, Pasini A et al.; Gruppo Italiano di Studio Endometriosi. Determinants of short term recurrence rate of endometriosis. Eur J Obstet Gynecol Reprod Biol 2005; 121: 216–19.

24. Weir E, Mustard C, Cohen M, Kung R. Endometriosis: what is the risk of hospital admission, readmission and major surgical inter-vention? J Minim Invasive Gynecol 2005; 12: 486–93.

25. Harrison RF, Barry-Kinsella C. Efficacy of medroxyprogesterone treatment in infertile women with endometriosis: a prospective, randomised, placebo-controlled study. Fertil Steril 2000; 74: 24–30.

26. Moen MH, Stockstad T. A long-term follow-up study of women with asymptomatic endometriosis diagnosed incidentally at sterilisation. Fertil Steril 2002; 78: 773–6.

CHAPTER 10

Ultrasound assessment of endometriosis

Bill Smith

INTRODUCTION

The role of ultrasound in the assessment of endometriosis has in the past been relatively limited. Conventional grey-scale two-dimensional (2D) scanning identified the formation of endometriotic cysts on the ovary but offered little indication as to the extent of the disease. Recent advances in scanning technology have, however, significantly enhanced the impact of ultrasound in diagnostic terms as well influencing clinical managements.

Improvements in grey-scale (G-S) imaging and colour Doppler imaging (CDI) sensitivity, the introduction and refinement of three-dimensional (3D) scanning and a more flexible approach to pelvic scanning have collectively increased the diagnostic capability of ultrasound techniques, particularly in this area of gynaecological investigation. Evidence of endometriosis and associated lesions can be detected at a much earlier stage, textural and vascular changes suggestive of adenomyosis recognised and the development of pelvic adhesions and other complications of the disease demonstrated with far greater certainty.

ULTRASOUND (GREY-SCALE) APPEARANCES OF ENDOMETRIOSIS

Improvements in transducer design and performance as well as new signal processing algorithms have resulted in higher-resolution G-S imaging. Developments such as compound resolution/focusing (CRI), speckle reduction (SRI) and harmonic (HI) imaging functions produce far greater tissue detail and the ability to visualise ovarian and pelvic lesions in the order of only a few millimetres size.

Figures 10.1–10.3 illustrate typical ultrasound (G-S) appearances of endometriotic cysts of the ovary. The cases also illustrate the level of ultrasound detail obtained from modern G-S systems (Figures 10.4 and 10.5).

The diagnosis of adenomyosis remains a particular issue from a medical imaging point of view. It is reasonable to say that, to date, magnetic resonance imaging (MRI) is regarded as perhaps the most effective modality in this respect, but presents obvious problems with regard to practical aspects and cost in particular. The availability of high-definition G-S imaging, as well as considerable advances in CDI techniques, has nevertheless had considerable impact in this respect. Diffuse myometrial thickening with irregular textural changes, enlargement of myometrial glands, poor differentiation of the myometrial-endometrial interface and, in particular, increased myometrial vascularity are all ultrasound features often found in cases of known endometriosis and/or confirmed adenomyosis.

SCANNING TECHNIQUES

Advances in transducer design and function afford a more flexible, comprehensive approach to scanning of the female pelvis. Any combination of transvaginal (TVS), transrectal (TRS) and transabdominal (TAS) scanning techniques can be readily utilised in order to fully evaluate an individual case of endometriosis. TVS remains the principal means for imaging of the pelvic organs and the essential component in the investigation of the disease and associated complications. Its ability to generate very high-definition G-S and CDI information of the body tissues is fully recognised and very widely documented.

TRS offers greater access and improved visualisation of the deep pelvis. It proves of particular benefit in cases of severe endometriosis, often presenting with extensive (bowel) adhesions and/or ovaries adherent towards the recto-uterine region. In these cases, TVS is sometimes poorly tolerated by the patient due to excessive discomfort on vaginal examination, and TRS usually provides a more appropriate alternative (Figure 10.8).

TAS cannot offer the image resolution expected of TVS techniques. Nevertheless, its wider field of view and the more penetrating ('lower frequency') ultrasound beam generated allows improved delineation of larger pelvic lesions. This is particularly beneficial in the assessment of large uterine fibroids as well as adenomyomas frequently found in cases of endometriosis. It also enables visualisation

(a)

(b)

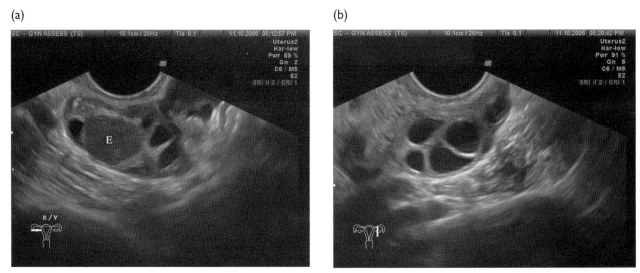

Figure 10.1 Combined use of harmonic imaging (HI), speckle reduction (SRI), compound resolution imaging (CRI) etc. very clearly delineates a single endometriotic cyst (E) of approximately 1 cm size only within the right ovary in (a). The lesion exhibits the characteristic homogenous G-S appearances which result from internal clotting of blood following sequential menstruation. Multiple immature follicles are very well outlined within both ovaries in (a) and (b) – this impression of increased follicular development and activity is apparent in many cases of endometriosis, particularly in the early stages of the disease

(a)

(b)

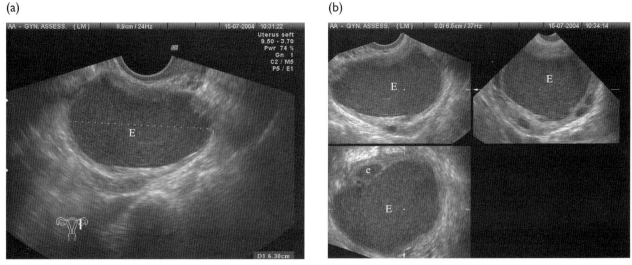

Figure 10.2 (a) This shows a large endometriotic cyst (E) again with its typical smooth grey-scale (G-S) appearance. (b) This is a multi-sectional 3D reconstruction of the same ovary and outlines the lesion (E) in parasagittal, transverse and coronal anatomical planes. Again they highlight the characteristic ultrasound features of this type of ovarian lesion. High-definition G-S imaging is able to identify a further, much smaller lesion (e) measuring less than 1 cm in size, shown within the coronal section. The sections also clearly delineate the presence of preserved, functional ovarian stroma with antral follicles evident

of (adherent) ovaries located towards the lateral and more superficial regions of the pelvic cavity.

COLOUR DOPPLER IMAGING

The increased sensitivity produced by the latest CDI systems provides valuable diagnostic information. Fine vascular (capillary) blood flow can be observed through most pelvic tissues and abnormal changes caused by gynaecological disease recognised more effectively. Hyperaemic changes

within the myometrium in particular can be clearly demonstrated (Figure 10.9). Increased myometrial vascularity appears to be a characteristic ultrasound feature noted in many cases of proven endometriosis, and certainly when the presence of adenomyosis is strongly suggested at clinical examination or confirmed at surgery.

Vascular changes within the ovarian stroma, usually accompanied by multifollicular development of the ovary, are again a very common feature identified in a significant number of cases. The formation of very active functional

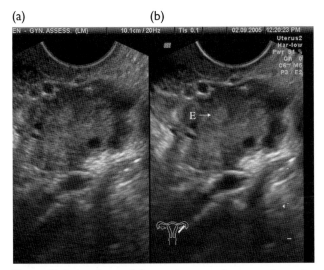

Figure 10.3 An adherent left ovary in a case of severe endometriosis. A composite image is shown of the same anatomical section utilising harmonic imaging (HI) in (a) but combined HI and speckle reduction imaging (SRI) in (b). An extremely small, probable endometrioma (E) of only a few millimetres size is visualised but with greater clarity by the additional use of SRI. Increased proliferation of ovarian stroma very often evident in cases of endometriosis is again demonstrated with greater clarity by SRI.

(ovulatory) cysts characterised by very prominent peripheral vascularity (angiogenesis) on CDI examination are often found on ultrasound assessment. This definite impression of increased ovarian (normal) activity might well explain the increased endometrial proliferation and development of polyps as well as the tendency for fibroid growth so often seen on ultrasound in patients with endometriosis.

Figure 10.7 again demonstrates the increased vascularity within the myometrium associated with adenomyosis. Figure 10.8 demonstrates the presence of an active ovulatory cyst, typically found in cases of endometriosis.

THREE-DIMENSIONAL ULTRASOUND

Tremendous advances in information technology (IT) capability have had considerable impact in ultrasound imaging generally, but especially so in the development of 3D scanning. Its clinical value has certainly been realised as part of gynaecological ultrasound and has proved of particular benefit in the assessment of endometriosis, gauging the extent of the disease and identifying complications arising from its presence.

Combined with modern transducer (TVS) technology, it provides increased, high-resolution anatomical information within the pelvis. Its principal advantage in diagnostic terms is the ability to obtain any anatomical plane within the body and to visualise the ultrasound information in the form of a multisectional display (See Figure 10.2b). 3D can involve other imaging formats (see 'Single Sweep Technology'), but from a practical and diagnostic point of view, multisectional displays remain the most useful in this area of medical ultrasound. 3D images can be viewed as a static format or in real-time (i.e. 4D ultrasound), but the latter offers little benefit in gynaecological applications.

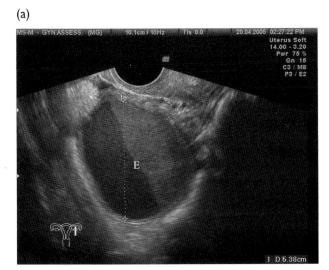
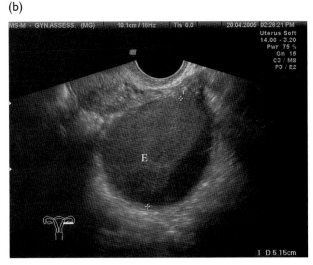

Figure 10.4 (a, b) Parasagittal and transverse sections demonstrating a large endometrioma of the ovary. A variation in the ultrasound greyscale (GS) appearances of the cyst compared to other examples shown is very evident. This has resulted from recent internal bleeding within the lesion associated with menstruation. Modern G-S imaging is able to differentiate between old clot and the fresh blood now contained. This can often give rise to a 'loculated' appearance to endometriotic cysts at this stage. The lesion resumes its characteristic G-S appearances once the fresh blood clots after a few days. Monitoring of these changes following menstruation is often useful in terms of differentiating between endometriotic cysts and other types of ovarian tumours (see Figure 10.5)

(a)

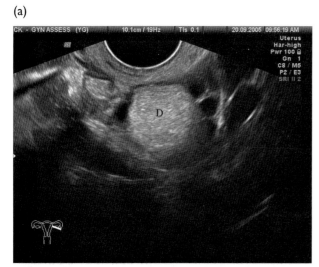

(b)

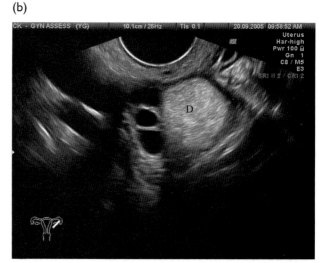

Figure 10.5 Ultrasound sections (a, b) through the ovary confirm the presence of a dermoid cyst (D). The dermoid is very clearly delineated, as well as multiple immature follicles, using combined harmonic (HI), speckle reduction (SRI), compound resolution (CRI) functions. Ultrasound features associated with lesions are nevertheless very similar to those of an endometrioma thereby causing uncertainty regarding the diagnosis. A post-menses scan within the first week of the menstrual cycle would, however, show no change at all in its ultrasound appearances. In the case of an endometrioma, the lesion would exhibit evidence of differential, internal haemorrhage as demonstrated in Figure 10.4 plus an increase in its size immediately following menstruation. The case serves to emphasise the benefit of a follow-up, post-menses scan assessment in terms of differentiating between endometriotic cysts and other types of ovarian lesions such as dermoids, luteal cysts, etc.

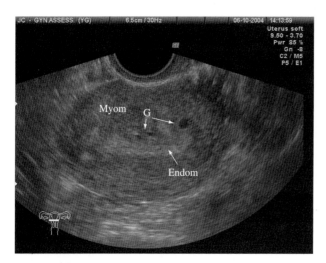

Figure 10.6 A transverse section through the uterus in a case of known adenomyosis. Grey-scale (G-S) imaging demonstrates an irregular, mottled appearance to the myometrium. There is definite loss of the anterior endometrial–myometrial interface. Prominent myometrial glands (G) are well demonstrated. The anterior uterine wall is thicker than the posterior wall and the uterus is generally enlarged in cross-section for a patient of this age (38 years) and nulliparity

Figures 10.10–10.12 demonstrate the value of the 3D TVS multisectional facility, including both G-S and CDI techniques. Figure 10.12 in particular highlights the diagnostic value of 3D multi-sectional displays in assessing complex features associated with severe, extensive endometriosis.

BLOOD PERFUSION STUDIES

In the past, the evaluation of tissue vascularity has been extremely limited and purely subjective in nature. Measurement of pelvic blood flow was restricted to spectral Doppler assessment of relatively major vessels. Very recent developments in 3D ultrasound technology have resulted in the combined utilisation of TVS–CDI–3D imaging formats to allow blood perfusion studies (BPS) of the pelvic organs.

BPS provide quantitative measurement of fine capillary blood flow through a given volume of tissue or individual pelvic structure. Blood flow indices are available which collectively reflect volume blood flow through tissues. The ability to quantify tissue vascularity in this way is becoming increasingly useful in recognising those changes associated with gynaecological disease. BPS readily identify and gauge increased vascularity within the pelvic tissues found in cases of endometriosis and especially those where adenomyosis is strongly suspected or proven to be present. This facility to investigate vascular changes within the myometrium and ovarian stroma in particular provides the means to confirm the likelihood of endometriosis at a very early stage of its development (Figure 10.13).

SINGLE SWEEP TECHNOLOGY

The introduction of 'Voluson Technology' has created a whole new concept in terms of 3D ultrasound imaging. A single, 5–10-second, electronically controlled sweep of the

(a)

(b)

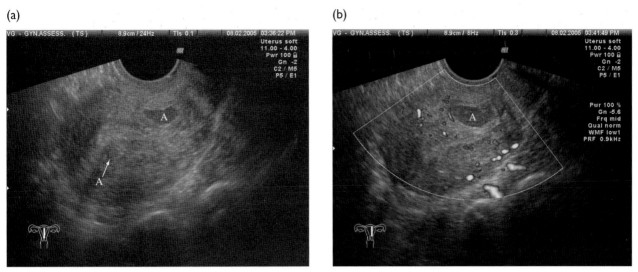

Figure 10.7 (a) This is a parasagittal section through the uterus showing irregular textural changes within the myometrium and a thickened posterior uterine wall. Evidence of two small developing adenomyomas (A) can be clearly delineated by high-resolution grey-scale (G-S) imaging. Poor differentiation of the myometrial–endometrial interface plus increased myometrial vascularity are demonstrated within a similar anatomical section in (b) and are further suggestive of adenomyosis

(a)

(b)

(c)

(d)

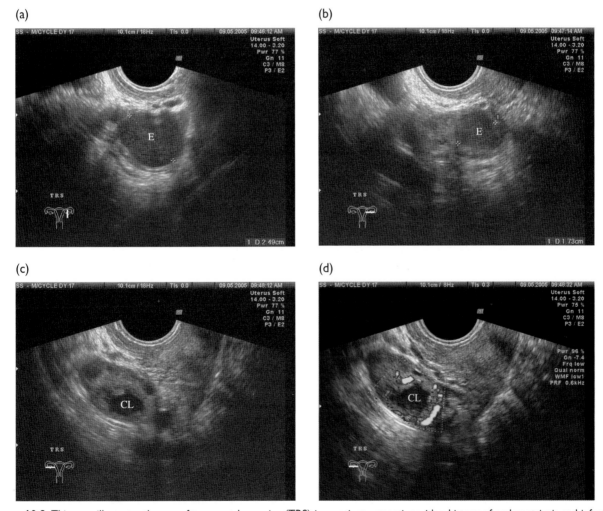

Figure 10.8 This case illustrates the use of transrectal scanning (TRS) in a patient presenting with a history of endometriosis and infertility. Both ovaries were adherent within the deep pelvis and poorly visualised by TVS. (a, b) These images clearly show a single endometrioma (E) measuring 2.1 cm in average diameter within the left ovary. Combined TRS–colour Doppler imaging (CDI) demonstrates an active corpus luteum (CL) within the right ovary: (c) TRS G-S imaging; (d) TRS–CDI

(a)

(b)   (c)

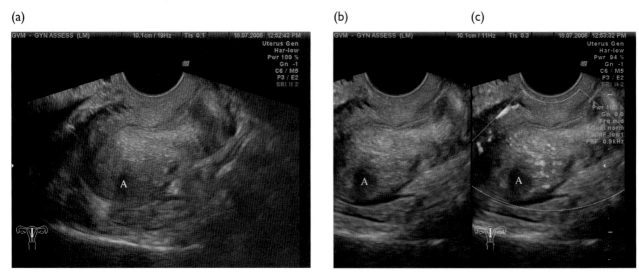

Figure 10.9 (a–c) Increased thickening of the posterior uterine wall is clearly visible. A single posterior wall adenomyoma (A) is demonstrated best in (b). Hyperaemic changes associated with diffuse adenomyosis are clearly shown by colour Doppler imaging (CDI) in (c)

ultrasound beam through the body tissues with the (TVS) transducer held stationary provides a wealth of anatomical and clinical information. The volumetric ultrasound data is stored instantaneously within the ultrasound machine. Ultrasound information can be rapidly retrieved and displayed, and the images manipulated as required within a few seconds. Figure 10.14 illustrates the different types of image formats which can be utilised in this respect.

The image formats displayed in Figure 10.14 greatly aid interpretation of scan information by the referring consultant. In cases of complex, extensive pathology, a clinical diagram to support the ultrasound images proves to be a considerable asset (Figure 10.11j).

Single sweep technology promotes post-scan evaluation and clinical reporting. It gives the confidence to review the ultrasound information after the completion of busy scan clinics without compromising the effectiveness of diagnostic evaluation at all. This proves particularly useful in the post-scan assessment of complex pelvic changes and adherent masses often associated with very severe cases of endometriosis. Scanning times and transducer movement are significantly reduced by applying single sweep scanning techniques to selected areas of pelvic cavity. Reduced scanning times are greatly appreciated by those patients experiencing extreme discomfort and considerable distress from conventional TVS techniques as a result of very extensive pelvic endometriosis.

Volumetric storage of image formation is very useful as an alternative to archiving large numbers of ultrasound pictures in the form of hard copies. It is also ideal for the purpose of retrieving previous images for comparison at later scans, particularly when following up cases of endometriosis. Further usefulness includes provision of material for educational/training programmes, etc. as well

as medicolegal aspects. Multi-sectional displays and tomographic ultrasound imaging (TUI) techniques are of particular value from the point of view of pre-surgical assessment and planning.

CLINICAL CASES

The following clinical cases reinforce the value of modern ultrasound scanning in the assessment of changes associated with endometriosis. They highlight the exceptional levels of diagnostic information state of the art ultrasound systems such as current GE Healthcare (Kretz) Voluson Technology have to offer.

Case 1: previous history of chronic pelvic and abdominal discomfort and menstrual issues – known history of grade I–II endometriosis

Images 1a and 1b show a persistent, haemorrhagic luteal cyst (C) on both ovaries. CDI investigation in Images 1c and 1d confirms increased activity of both lesions. TVS assessment of the uterus in Images 1e and 1f shows G-S and CDI changes suggestive of adenomyosis – localised increased myometrial vascularity might well be associated with the development of an adenomyoma (A). The case emphasises the ovarian activity and vascular changes which often give rise to symptoms in early stages of the disease.

Case 2: previous history of pelvic pain and menstrual irregularity

Images 2a and 2b show textural irregularity and increased vascularity of the myometrium suggestive of adenomyosis. The uterus is rotationally displaced but TVS G-S shows a thickened, polypoidal endometrium – CDI excludes 'high-risk' changes. Images 2c and 2d demonstrate a developing fibroid (M) within the right upper uterine wall – CDI

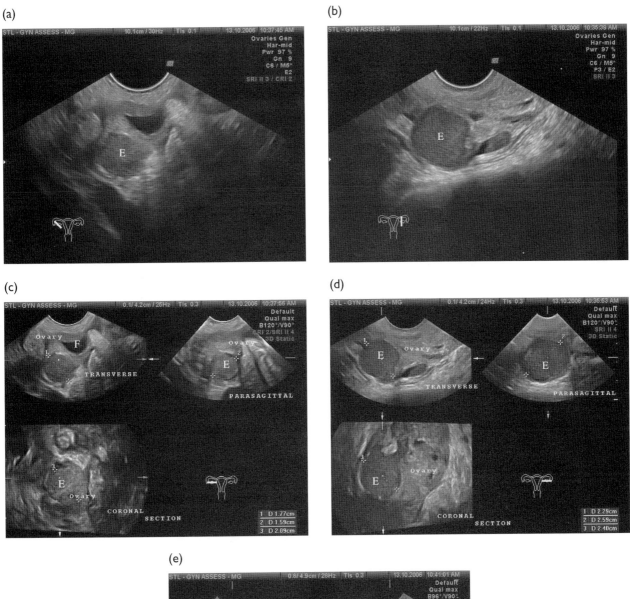

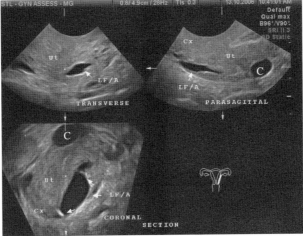

Figure 10.10 (a,b) An endometriotic cyst (E) is identified on both ovaries on transvaginal scanning (TVS) assessment. Multisectional 3D reconstruction of planes through both ovaries, respectively, delineates the lesion (E) on each side with greater precision, provides more accurate measurement of their sizes and clearly demonstrates normal ovarian tissue (c,d). A follicular cyst (F) is partly seen on the right ovary in (c). (e) Multisectional displays can be further manipulated to demonstrate the extent of loculated fluid/adhesions (LF/A) to the left lower posterolateral aspect of the uterus. A further simple pelvic (fimbrial) cyst (C) was identified

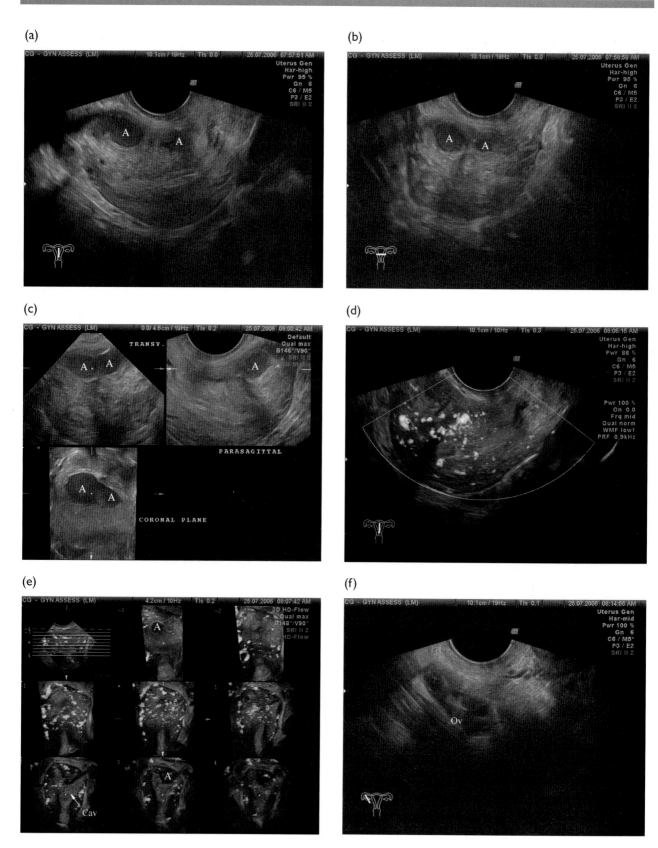

Continued

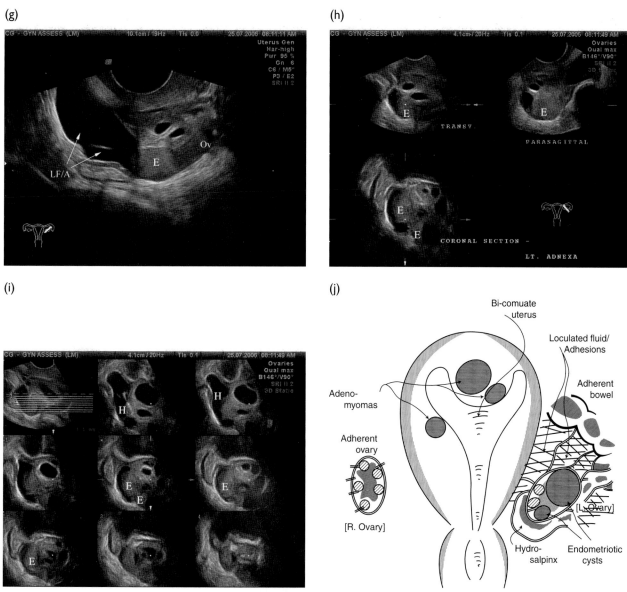

Figure 10.11 (a,b) Parasagittal and transverse 2D transvaginal scanning (TVS) sections through the uterus. Grey-scale (G-S) appearances confirm the presence of two adenomyomas (A) within the anterior uterine wall. 3D multisectional displays are shown in (c) which confirm the location and extent of the lesions with much more precision. (d) This demonstrates increased myometrial vascularity characteristic of adenomyosis. (e) This confirms the same vascular changes using multi-sectional tomographic imaging (TUI) format in the coronal plane – the adenomyomas (A), endometrial cavity (Cav) and myometrial vascularity are clearly visualised in these MRI type tomographic images. (f) This shows an adherent right ovary (Ov). (g) This shows an adherent left ovary (Ov) containing an endometriotic cyst (E) – paraovarian loculated fluid collections and adhesions (LF/A) are clearly delineated within the left adnexal region using 2D G-S imaging. (h,i) This are multisectional 3D and TVS displays giving much more anatomical information within the left adnexal region. A further smaller endometriotic cyst (E) is confirmed, and the multi-follicular nature of the ovary is shown with far greater clarity. The extent of adnexal loculated fluid/adhesions is again shown with greater precision, and the presence of the left hydrosalpinx (H) confirmed following post-scan manipulation of TUI views. (j) Clinical Diagrams are of tremendous value as part of ultrasound scan reports i.e. to support the ultrasound images. This is particularly so in the reporting of complex pelvic findings where extensive endometriosis and associated complications might be present. This example relates to the case imaged in (a–c) and the sketch involved greatly enhances clinical communication for the referring clinician

confirms an established vascular supply to the lesion. Two anterior wall adenomyomas (A) are also clearly seen. The development of endometrial polyps and uterine fibroids is a frequent feature associated with the presence of endometriosis and probably reflects increased ovarian

(hormonal) activity usually evident even within early stages of the disease. Images 2e and 2f confirm the presence of an active, haemorrhagic corpus luteum (CL) on the right ovary. TVS, G-S and CDI techniques in Images 2g and 2h confirm the typical ultrasound appearance of an

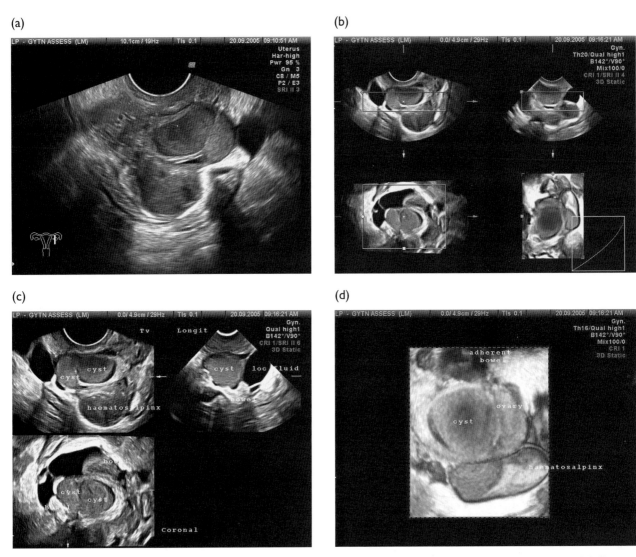

Figure 10.12 (a) This shows a complex, adherent mass within the left adnexa using conventional transvaginal grey-scale (TVS G-S) imaging. The use of multisectional displays in (b) to include surface rendering (ST) enhancement identifies individual components and structures within the tissue mass. Further manipulation of multisectional images in (c) demonstrates endometriotic cysts within the left ovary, with paraovarian loculated fluid collections and adhesions involving both bowel and ovary. The enhanced ST image in (d) clearly delineates a haematosalpinx adherent to and wrapped around the ovary with adherent bowel again demonstrated

endometrioma (E) within the left ovary. No significant peripheral vascularity is shown by CDI around the lesion – this is characteristic of the vast majority of endometriotic cysts, although not all, and helps differentiate them from haemorrhagic functional (ovulatory) cysts as seen on the right ovary in this case. Multisectional and TUI displays as shown in Images 2i and 2j respectively delineate the lesion (E) with greater clarity and provide detailed imaging of a probably adherent left ovary.

Case 3: previous history of heavy, painful periods – known history of endometriosis

Image 3a shows diffuse, excessive thickening of the posterior uterine wall with very poor differentiation between myometrium and irregular, thickened endometrial tissue.

G-S appearances are consistent with extensive adenomyosis. CDI changes in Image 3b show increased myometrial vascularity and confirm the diagnosis.

Case 4: previous history of endometriosis – attending for hysterosonosalpingiography (HSS/'HyCoSy') assessment of the fallopian tubes

Diagnosis: demonstration of myometrial gland proliferation associated with extensive adenomyosis

Image 4a shows typical TVS G-S changes within the posterior uterine wall, very suggestive of adenomyosis immediately prior to the procedure. The tip (T) of the catheter and distended catheter balloon (B) fixing it in place are identified in Image 4b. Image 4c is a parasagittal section of the uterus/uterine cavity showing flow of the contrast

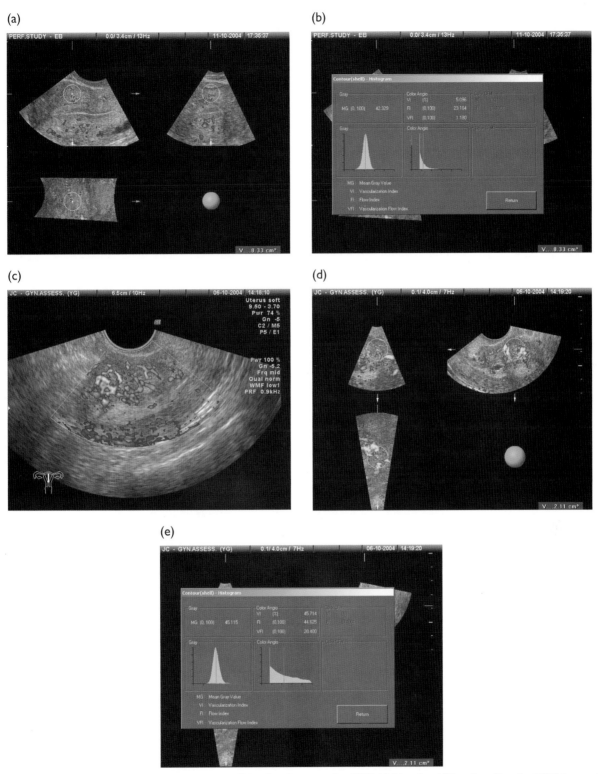

Figure 10.13 These cases demonstrate the principles of blood perfusion studies (BPS). Multisectional 3D–colour Doppler (CDI) images show myometrial vascularity within a 'normal' case in (a) – a 'sphere' has been used in this example to isolate a volume of myometrial tissue in three planes. (b) This displays the 'blood flow indices' (VI, FI, VFI), and their values confirm normal levels of vascularity. (c) This demonstrates a CDI parasagittal section through the uterus in a known case of adenomyosis – increased myometrial vascularity is clearly shown. (d) This shows similar placement of the sample volume to that in (a). A significant variation in the values of blood flow indices is obvious in (e), consistent with hyperaemic changes associated with endometriosis (adenomyosis). Volume samples can be varied in size, shape, etc. and accurately reselected in terms of their location using multisectional 3D imaging. The use of BPS is in its early stages of development, and technical issues relating particularly to the reproducibility of results remain. Nevertheless they provide a means of quantifying tissue vascularity, and experience shows increasing reliability in identifying and measuring abnormal changes, particularly those associated with endometriosis

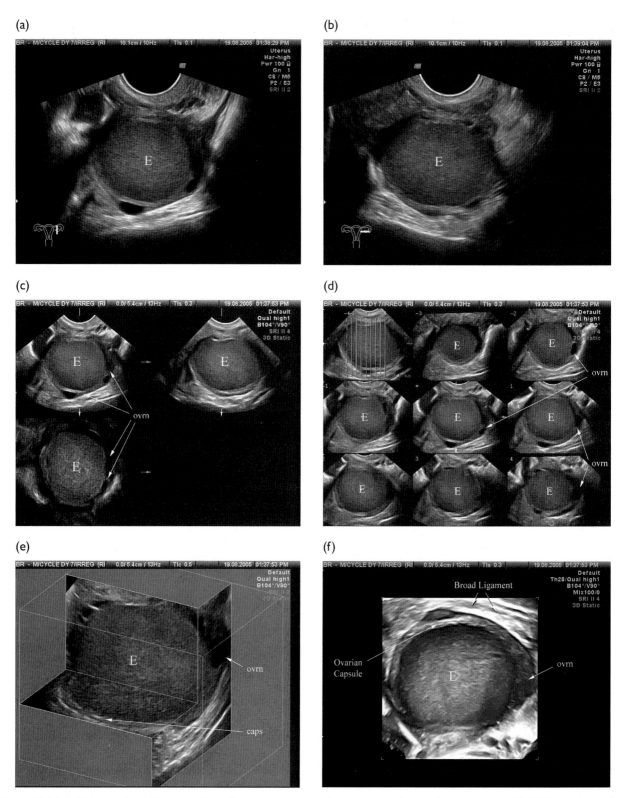

Figure 10.14 (a,b) Conventional 2D parasaggital and transverse sections demonstrating a large endometriotic cyst (E). (c) This is the resulting multisectional display clearly delineating the size and extent of the lesion with greater precision, and confirms the presence of functional ovarian tissue (ovrn) with antral follicles stretched over the endometrioma (E). These findings are further confirmed by multisectional tomographic imaging (TUI, transverse plane), clearly showing preserved, normal ovarian tissue (ovrn) in (d). (e) This illustrates the ability to display block volumes again useful to highlight the capsule of the lesion (caps) and normal ovarian tissue (ovrn). (f) This is a surface rerdered (ST) image of the endometrioma and provides enhanced visualisation of the lesion and preserved, normal ovarian tissue. These imaging formats give extremely precise ultrasound information with recognisable anatomical planes to send to referring consultants as part of the scan report. They provide valuable preoperative information and considerably improved levels of clinical communication

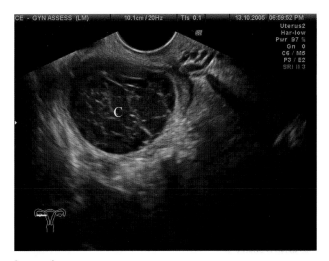

Image 1a

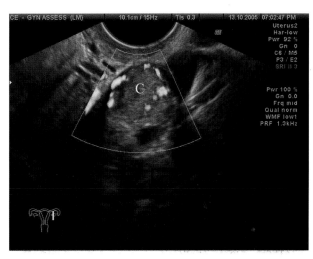

Image 1d

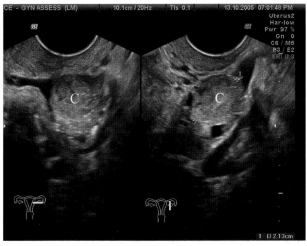

Image 1b

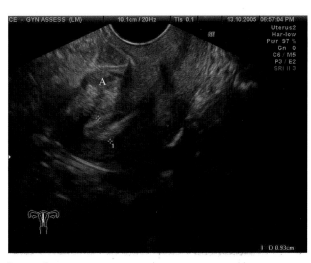

Image 1e

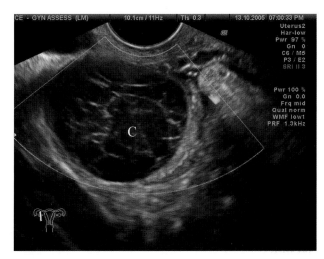

Image 1c

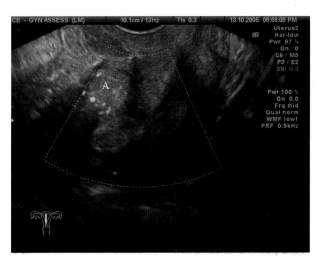

Image 1f

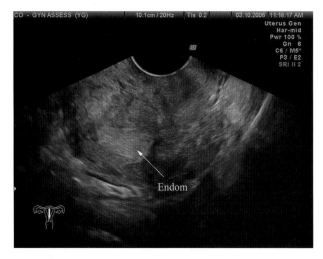

Image 2a

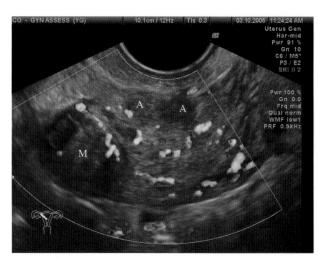

Image 2d

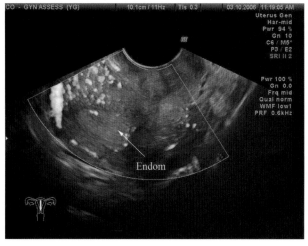

Image 2b

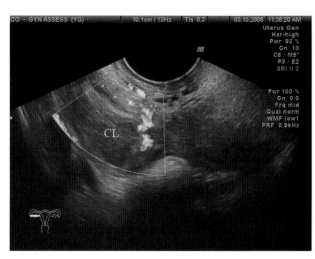

Image 2e

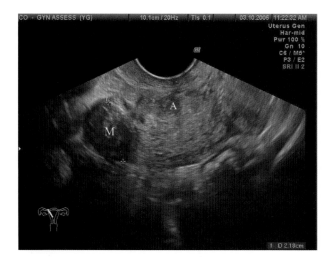

Image 2c

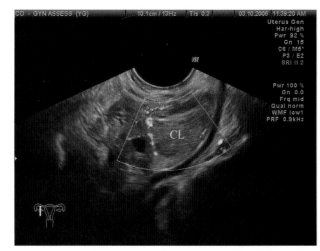

Image 2f

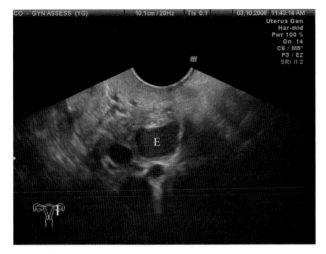

Image 2g

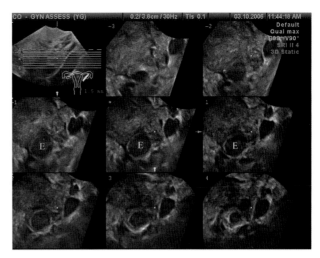

Image 2j

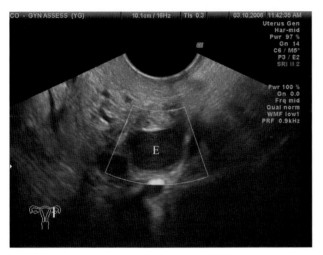

Image 2h

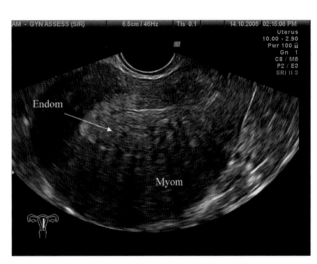

Image 3a

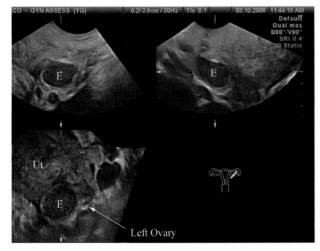

Image 2i

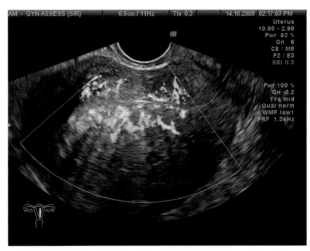

Image 3b

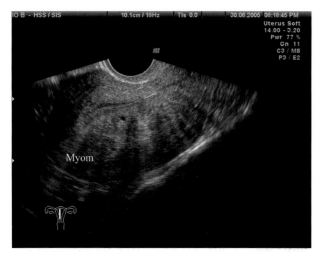

Image 4a

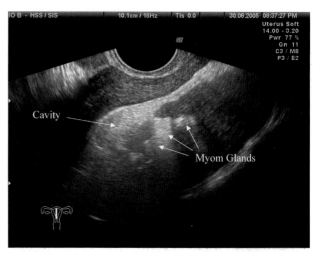

Image 4d

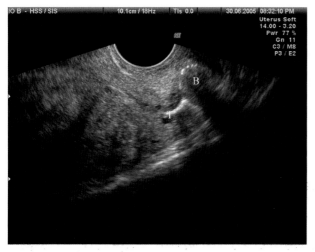

Image 4b

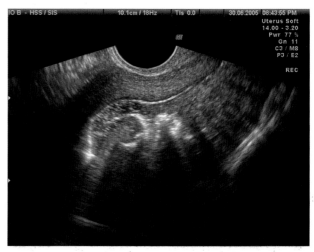

Image 4e

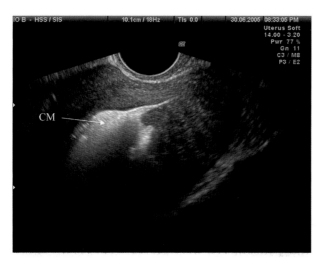

Image 4c

medium (CM) into the mid-upper cavity. Image 4d shows the cavity very clearly, but confirms free flow of the contrast medium into enlarged myometrial glands. The procedure was halted, and passive emptying of the contrast medium from the glands back into the cavity is observed in Image 4e. HSS confirmed proliferation of myometrial glands in a case of very severe adenomyosis.

Case 5: previous history of abdominal discomfort – known history of extensive endometriosis

Diagnosis: endometriosis associated with umbilical adhesions

The images are all TAS: Images 5a and 5d were carried out using a conventional transabdominal transducer; Images 5b, 5c, 5e and 5f were carried out using a high-resolution 'breast probe' in order to achieve increased ultrasound detail within the superficial tissues of the abdomen.

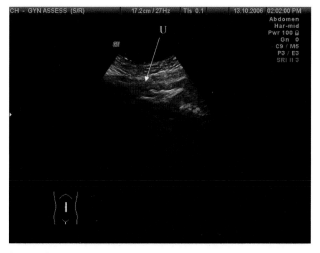

Image 5a

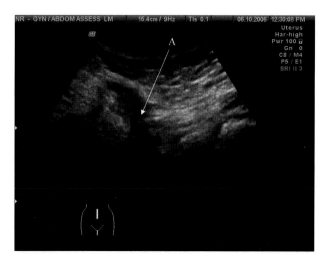

Image 5d

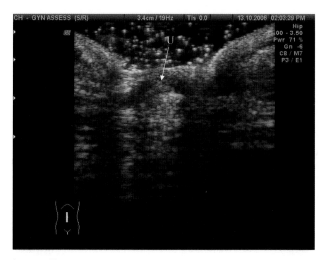

Image 5b

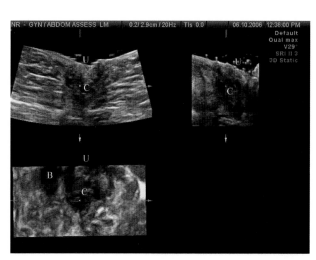

Image 5e

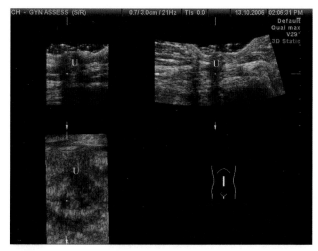

Image 5c

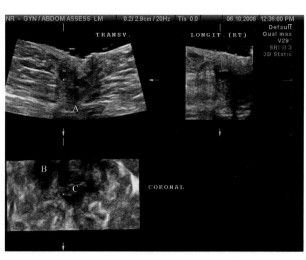

Image 5f

Images 5a–5c show 'normal' appearances from another patient for comparison purposes. No significant features associated with the umbilicus (U) or underlying tissues were noted. The presence of clot (C) underlying the umbilicus within the affected case is very obvious. An area of more recent haemorrhage (B) was noted and probably reflects menstrual bleeding from endometriotic tissue present with an obvious adhesion (A) between bowel and the anterior abdominal wall. The finding explained cyclical bleeding from the umbilicus during the post-menses phase of the cycle.

Case 6: previous history of severe pelvic pain – known history of extensive endometriosis

Diagnosis: rectovaginal endometriosis

Images 6a and 6b are parasagittal sections of the uterus showing textural irregularities and significantly increased thickening of the posterior wall of a retroverted uterus. Localised vascular changes were demonstrated by CDI, shown in Image 6c. G-S and CDI appearances are consistent with adenomyosis. An adenomyoma (A) is noted within the posterior uterine wall. It should be noted that a very high proportion of patients with endometriosis present with a retroverted uterus! Images 6d and 6e show typical multifollicular change and increased stromal development in both ovaries. Image 6f confirms the presence of a very active corpus luteum on the left ovary as confirmed by CDI. TVS–CDI assessment of the rectovaginal septum confirms an abnormal increase in tissue vascularity within that area in Image 6g. 3D TUI parasagittal sections in Image 6h show a clear demarcation and separation between the vagina (V) and rectum (R) towards one side. The interface is lost and obvious adhesions involving the vaginal and rectal walls can be visualised in image slices within the mid-line region and moving towards the opposite side. The combination of

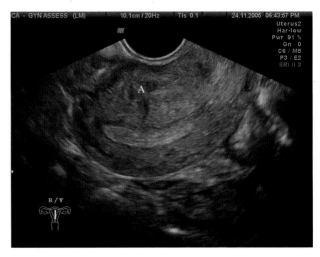

Image 6b

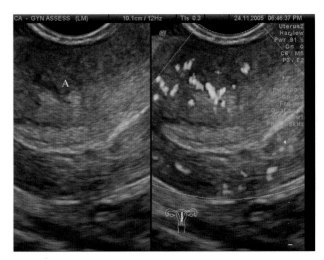

Image 6c

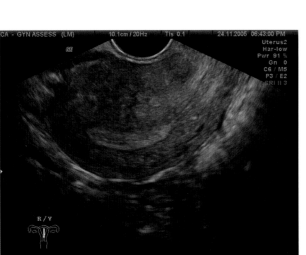

Image 6a

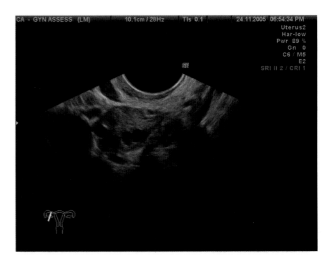

Image 6d

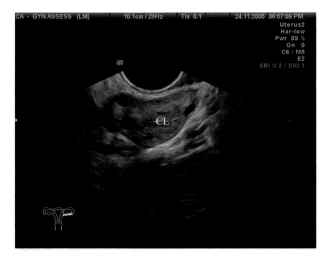

Image 6e

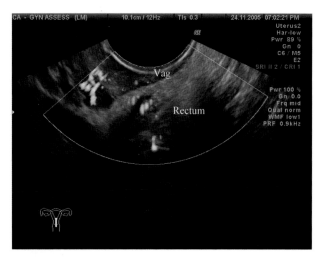

Image 6g

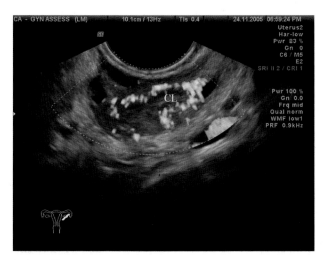

Image 6f

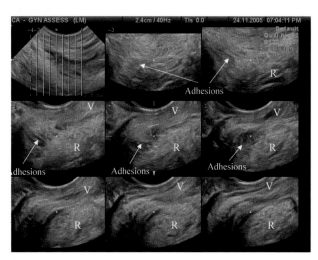

Image 6h

high-resolution 3D TVS imaging and CDI confirms extensive rectovaginal adhesions associated with pelvic endometriosis and likely endometriosis associated with the rectovaginal region.

CONCLUSIONS

1. Ultrasound techniques have a crucial role to play in the investigation of endometriosis and the assessment of those patients experiencing clinical symptoms which could be suggestive of the disease.

2. Modern ultrasound imaging has the capacity to identify anatomical and vascular features associated with very early stages of the disease in a significant number of cases. The formation of endometriotic cysts of the ovary confirming the presence of the disease can be visualised at a very early stage of development.

3. Advances in ultrasound technology have had a major impact in the detection of endometriosis as well as gauging the extent of the disease and confirming secondary complications arising from its presence. Ultrasound scanning in this area of gynaecology requires the latest in 2D and 3D G-S imaging and CDI techniques. A comprehensive, flexible approach to scanning is essential to fully investigate all cases in which the disease is suspected.

4. CDI/BPS techniques combined with high-resolution G-S capability are able to confirm the probability of adenomyosis with increasing certainty.

5. Single sweep (Voluson) technology provides tremendous benefits in diagnostic terms and the facility for accurate post-scan evaluation of cases. In addition it offers new concepts in the manipulation and transfer of ultrasound

data, storage of image information, improved levels of reporting and more effective clinical communication.

6. The latest ultrasound systems such as the GE Healthcare (Kretz) Voluson range and new developments in scanning techniques provide an extremely reliable, convenient and very cost effective means of investigating endometriosis. Scanning remains safe and well tolerated from the patients' perspective. Modern technology has established ultrasound as the principal modality for the detection of endometriosis, particularly in the early stages of the disease, and has had considerable impact in terms of clinical managements.

CHAPTER 11

Nutrition and endometriosis

Marilyn Glenville

The focus of the nutritional approach to endometriosis is to reduce pain, lower oestrogen levels, improve liver function, control prostaglandin production to lower inflammation, increase sex hormone binding globulin (SHBG) and improve immune function.

The nutritional treatment is a combination of dietary and supplement recommendations together with general suggestions for stress reduction and lifestyle changes.

DIETARY MODIFICATIONS

Diet has been shown to modify the risk of a number of oestrogen-related cancers such as endometrial[1], breast[2] and ovarian cancer[3], so dietary modifications have been investigated in relation to oestrogen-dependent endometriosis.

Diets high in saturated fat increase concentrations of serum oestrogen[4], and women who ate meat once a day were up to twice as likely to have endometriosis compared to those who ate less red meat and more fruit and vegetables[5]. The women who had the highest intake of red meat increased their risk of endometriosis by between 80 and 100%. The women with the highest intake of fresh fruit and vegetables lowered their risk of endometriosis by about 40%.

Phytoestrogens such as flax (linseed) can help to reduce circulating levels of oestrogen. Flaxseed, the richest known source of plant lignans (one type of phytoestrogen), has been shown to have a modulating effect on oestrogen metabolism. Two competing pathways in oestrogen metabolism involve the 2-hydroxylated and 16α-hydroxylated metabolites. The balance of the two metabolites has been used as a marker of breast cancer risk. Over two menstrual cycles, women ate their usual diet plus baked goods containing either 10 g of flaxseed, 28 g of wheat bran, 10 g of flaxseed plus 28 g of wheat bran or no flaxseed or wheat bran. The addition of flaxseed increased the urinary 2 : 16 α-hydroxyestrone ratio but wheat bran had no effect. It is suggested that flaxseed may have a chemoprotective effect for women, but this may also be relevant to endometriosis, which is an oestrogen-dependent condition[6].

One possible mechanism underlying dysmenorrhoea is a disturbed balance between anti-inflammatory, vasodilatory eicosanoids derived from omega 3 fatty acids and pro-inflammatory, vasoconstrictor eicosanoids derived from omega 6 fatty acids[7]. In one study, menstrual pain was highly significantly correlated with a low intake of marine *n*-3 fatty acids[8]. *Trans* fatty acids (made from vegetable oils in a process called hydrogenation and found in margarines and baked goods, etc.) inhibit the enzyme Δ^6-desaturase, which is needed for the conversion of omega 3 fatty acids into anti-inflammatory prostaglandins. These *trans* fats also reduce the fluidity of cell membranes and have a negative effect on the structure of nerve and brain cells as well as interfering with the formation of anti-inflammatory prostaglandins (Figure 11.1).

A diet omitting caffeine and sugar and supplementing with essential fatty acids resulted in the authors of one study commenting that 'correction of the biochemical imbalance of the eicosanoid system and the hypersecretion of insulin that results from excessive intake of glycaemic carbohydrates and lack of essential fatty acids significantly decreases symptoms in patients with endometriosis and associated neuromuscular disease of the gastrointestinal tract'[9]. Controlling blood glucose is crucial with endometriosis, as higher levels of insulin cause the liver to produce less SHBG.

Red meat and dairy produce both contain arachidonic acid, which encourages the production of the pro-inflammatory prostaglandin PGE_2.

SHBG has been shown to be increased by a low-fat vegetarian diet. Thirty-three women followed a low-fat, vegetarian diet for two menstrual cycles. In a crossover design, they then followed their usual diet and took a placebo supplement. The low-fat vegetarian diet was associated with significant increases in SHGB and reductions in dysmenorrhoea duration and intensity and premenstrual symptom duration. The researchers suggested that the symptom change may be due to the dietary influences on oestrogen activity[10]. Lignans in flaxseed can also increase SHBG[11].

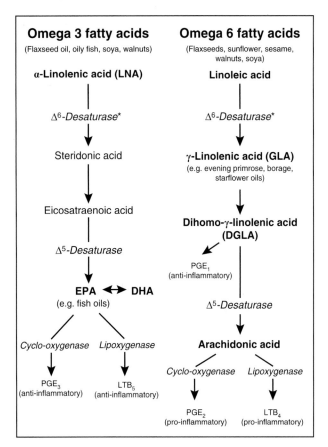

Figure 11.1 The metabolic pathways of the major *trans* fatty acids. *Factors thought to impair Δ^6-desaturase activity include Mg, Zn and B_6 deficiency; aging; alcohol; *trans* fatty acids; and high cholesterol levels. DHA, docosahexaenoic acid; EPA, eicosapentaenoic acid; LTB, leukotriene B; PGE, prostaglandin.

SUPPLEMENTS

It has become apparent that women are not getting everything they need from a 'well-balanced' diet. The National Diet and Nutrition Survey[12] showed that 84% of women fail to achieve the Reference Nutrient Intake (RNI replaced the Recommended Daily Allowance (RDA)) for folic acid, leading to the proposal that bread should be fortified with this vitamin. Some 74% failed to achieve the RNI for magnesium, 45% for zinc and 15% for vitamin D.

Overall, 74% of women are falling short on nutrients from their diet, with an 80% decrease in the consumption of omega 3 fatty acids[13]. In general, even with all the UK government messages, only 15% of women and 13% of men actually eat the five-a-day target for fruit and vegetables.

The other factor to consider is that even with the best intentions, the nutritional content of modern-day food is lacking. With the dominance of supermarket shopping, there is no way of knowing the freshness or nutritional content of food. A Consumer *Which?* Report in 2004 found that packs of sliced green beans contained only 11% of the

vitamin C they should have. The independent Food Commission's *Food Magazine* highlighted in 2005 that, comparing fruits and vegetables from the 1930s to the 1980s, modern fruits and vegetables were depleted in minerals by an average of 20%, and the magnesium levels of 27 vegetables had dropped by 24%, calcium by 46%, iron by 27% and zinc by 59%. This year (2006) the Food Commission looked at the mineral content of meat and dairy, comparing the 1930s to the most recent government tables, published in 2002. The mineral depletion overall was considerable, with the iron content in meat items having fallen on average by 47% and some products with a fall of 80%. The iron content of milk products dropped by over 60%, and copper and magnesium showed losses in meat products and dairy foods. Calcium loss from milk was only slight, but with cheeses it averaged over 15%, and in Parmesan cheese the loss was 70%.

Antioxidants

It has been suggested that in the presence of oxidative stress, reactive oxygen species might increase the growth and adhesion of endometrial cells. In one study, endometrial stromal cells from women with and without endometriosis were subjected to antioxidants or agents inducing oxidative stress. The authors concluded that 'increased oxidative stress and depletion of antioxidants may contribute to excessive growth of endometrial stromal cells'[14]. Another recent study has confirmed that oxidative stress might play a role in the development of endometriosis[15]. A good review article in 2005 suggested that oxidative stress can influence the entire reproductive lifespan of a woman and have a role to play in pathological processes involving the female reproductive system, including endometriosis[16]. Women with endometriosis have lower antioxidant intakes of vitamin C, vitamin E, selenium and zinc than do controls, and as endometriosis severity intensifies, an even lower intake of antioxidants is present[17]. Vitamin E can help to reduce dysmenorrhoea and also reduce blood loss[18].

Antioxidant-rich foods should be an important dietary focus for women with endometriosis, and antioxidant supplements should be included for around 3 months to enhance this effect.

It has been suggested that cell-mediated immunity in women with endometriosis may be decreased[19], with a lowering in the capacity of monocytes to mediate cytolysis of the misplaced endometrial cells and increased resistance of these cells to apoptosis. Decreased spontaneous apoptosis in women with endometriosis has been confirmed in a number of studies, and can result in the abnormal survival of endometrial cells allowing them to proliferate and implant[20,21]. Most of the antioxidant nutrients, including zinc and vitamin C, will help to support the normal functioning of the immune system, so these are important nutrients in the nutritional treatment protocol for endometriosis.

Omega 3 fatty acids

Not only are the omega 3 fatty acids important for their anti-inflammatory effects, but DHA (docosahexaenoic acid) causes decreased binding of oestradiol to oestrogen receptors[22]. Supplementation of omega 3 fatty acids, particularly fish oil, is important, as many women will follow no-fat or low-fat diets, and there are concerns that the consumption of foods containing omega 3 fatty acids is not adequate. Zinc, magnesium and vitamin B_6 are also needed for the correct metabolism of essential fatty acids into anti-inflammatory prostaglandins (PGE_1 and PGE_3).

In vitro studies show that a high omega 3 : 6 fatty acid ratio significantly reduces the survival of endometrial cells from women with and without endometriosis, and omega 3 fatty acids 'may be useful in the management of endometriosis by reducing the inflammatory response and modulating cytokine function'[23].

The liver conjugates oestrogens to their less active forms, which are then excreted in the bile into the intestines, and these conjugated oestrogens are excreted in the faeces. However, the conjugated oestrogens can be activated by the enzyme β-glucoronidase, which can deconjugate an oestrogen and recirculate it. The balance of the gut flora is therefore an important part of the nutritional treatment protocol for endometriosis, as probiotics can lower faecal β-glucuronidase activity, lower deconjugation of hormones in the colon and prevent their enteropathic resorption. Flaxseed can also help to remove endogenous oestrogen via increased retention in the gut for elimination in the faeces[24].

B vitamins

The B vitamins (B_6, B_{12} and folic acid) are involved in oestrogen conjugation and methylation, and vitamin B_1 can help with dysmenorrhoea. In one study, 556 women with moderate to severe dysmenorrhoea were given vitamin B_1 (100 mg per day) first for 90 days, and then changed to a placebo. Others were given the placebo first for 90 days and the B_1 next. Some 87% were 'completely cured', 8% were relieved and 5% showed no effect. The effect remained for at least 2 months after the B_1 was stopped. The authors commented: 'unlike all the current treatments which are suppression-oriented, this curative treatment directly treats the cause, is free from side effects, is inexpensive and easy to administer'[25].

Low intakes of vitamin B_{12} are coincident with a low omega 3 : 6 ratio[8].

Magnesium

Magnesium is known for its relaxing effects on muscle tissue, and can help with dysmenorrhoea and lower back pain[26]. Magnesium also increases the activity of glucuronyl transferase, an enzyme involved in hepatic glucuronidation, so is important for oestrogen detoxification.

LIFESTYLE

As well as the dietary and supplement recommendations, two lifestyle factors need to be taken into account with the treatment of endometriosis.

Stress

The modern lifestyle creates stress in the shape of traffic jams, late trains, missed appointments, financial worries work and family, and apart from its more general effects on health, it can have a role in endometriosis.

The enzyme Δ^6-desaturase comes into play to convert α-linolenic acid (ALA) to eicosapentaenoic acid (EPA), and this enzyme is reduced by stress, so less of the anti-inflammatory prostaglandins are produced. But at the same time, stress increases the conversion of dihomo-γ-linolenic acid (DGLA) to arachidonic acid, which in turn produces the pro-inflammatory prostaglandins.

Xenoestrogens

Some oestrogen exposure is exogenous through environmental oestrogens and xenoestrogens, from the pesticide and plastics industries. Male fish can express female characteristics, and a 5-year study by the Environment Agency (July 2006) showed that half the male fish in English rivers are developing female characteristics. These endocrine-disrupting chemicals can also influence human development, and possibly play a role in uterine disease such as endometriosis and fibroids[27].

Research has shown an association between dioxins and the development of endometriosis. Some 79% of female rhesus monkeys spontaneously developed endometriosis after being fed food containing dioxins, and the severity of the endometriosis was dose-related[28]. Dioxins can be found in food, but are also a by-product of chlorine-bleaching process paper and pulp mills, so it is recommended that women with endometriosis use organic cotton sanitary towels and tampons.

SUMMARY

The link between nutrition and health has been known for centuries. Around 400BC, Hippocrates wrote in depth on this subject, and in 1747, Dr James Lind observed that citrus fruits containing vitamin C could cure scurvy. In animal husbandry, the use of nutrition and nutritional supplements for reproduction and pregnancy is widely recognised. However, even in this era of modern medicine, the link between nutrient intake and health is not fully acknowledged, as well as that many diseases (e.g. cardiovascular disease[29], age-related macular degeneration[30] and insulin resistance[31]) could be treated or prevented by the correct use of dietary and nutrient intervention.

It is important that women with endometriosis know about the scientific advances in the role of nutrition in controlling and alleviating the symptoms of endometriosis.

Dietary recommendations

- reduction of foods that are high in saturated fats
- increase of foods rich in unsaturated fats, such as olive oil, nuts, seeds and oily fish
- organic foods wherever possible, to avoid ingesting higher levels of xenoestrogens and other unacceptable chemicals used in the growing or preserving process
- eliminating caffeine, including that found in tea, colas, coffee and chocolate
- weight control, as excess weight can lead to higher oestrogen levels
- reduced alcohol intake in order to improve liver detoxification of oestrogen
- regular exercise, which can help to decrease pain.

Supplement programme

- a multivitamin and mineral supplement
- B complex vitamins (50 mg of each B vitamin per day)
- magnesium (300 mg per day)
- vitamin E (300 iu per day)
- zinc citrate (15 mg per day)
- vitamin C with bioflavonoids (1000 mg twice per day)
- fish oil (1000 mg per day)
- probiotic.

Note that each nutrient represents the total intake per day, so if the multivitamin and mineral contains 100 mg then additional magnesium supplement only needs to contain 200 mg.

REFERENCES

1. Ta MH, Xu WH, Zheng W et al. A case-controlled study in Shanghai of fruit and vegetable intake and endometrial cancer. Br J Cancer 2005; 92: 2059–64.

2. Colomer R, Menendez JA. Mediterranean diet, olive oil and cancer. Clin Transl Oncol 2006; 8: 15–21.

3. Kiania F, Knutsen S, Singh P et al. Dietary risk factors for ovarian cancer: the Adventist Health Study (US). Cancer Causes Control 2006; 17: 137–46.

4. Nagata C, Takatsuka N, Kawakami N et al. Total and monounsaturated fat intake and serum oestrogen concentrations in premenopausal Japanese women. Nutr Cancer 2000; 38: 37–9.

5. Parazzini F, Chiaffarino F, Surace M et al. Selected food intake and risk of endometriosis. Hum Reprod 2004; 19: 1755–59.

6. Haggans CJ, Travelli EJ, Thomas W et al. The effect of flaxseed and wheat bran consumption on urinary estrogen metabolites in premenopausal women. Cancer Epidemiol Biomarkers Prev 2000; 9: 719–25.

7. Saldeen P, Saldeen T. Women and omega-3 fatty acids. Obstet Gynecol Surv 2004; 59i: 722–30.

8. Deutch B. Menstrual pain in Danish women correlated with low n-3 polyunsaturated fatty acid intake. Eur J Clin Nutr 1995; 49: 508–16.

9. Mathias R, Franklin R, Quast DC et al. Relation of endometriosis and neuromuscular disease of the gastrointestinal tract: new insights. Fertil Steril 1998; 70: 81–8.

10. Barnard ND, Scialli AR, Hurlock D, Bertron P. Diet and sex-hormone binding globulin, dysmenorrhoea and premenstrual syndrome. Obstet Gynecol 2000; 95: 245–50.

11. Haggans CJ, Hutchins AM, Olson BA et al. Effect of flaxseed consumption on urinary oestrogen metabolites in postmenopausal women. Nutr Cancer 1999; 33: 188–95.

12. Hoare J, Henderson, L, Bates CJ et al. The National Diet and Nutrition Survey: adults aged 19–64 years. 2005; Volume 5: Summary Report. London: HMSO, 2005.

13. Simopoulos AO. Omega 3 fatty acids in health and disease and in growth and development. Am J Clin Nutr 1991; 54: 438–63.

14. Fovouzi N, Berkkanoglu M, Arici A et al. Effect of oxidants and anti-oxidants on proliferation of endometrial stromal cells. Fertil Steril 2004; 82 (Suppl 3): 1019–22.

15. Jackson LW, Schistermann EF, Dev-Rao R et al. Oxidative stress and endometriosis. Hum Reprod 2005; 20: 2014–20.

16. Agarwal A, Gupta S, Sharma RK. Role of oxidative stress in female reproduction. Reprod Biol Endocrinol 2005; 14: 3–28.

17. Hernandez Guerrero CA, Bujalil Montenegro L, de la Jara Diaz J et al. Endometriosis and deficient intake of antioxidants molecules related to peripheral and peritoneal oxidative stress. Ginecol Obstet Mex 2006; 74: 20–8.

18. Ziaei S, Sakeri M, Kazemnejad A. A randomised controlled trial of vitamin E in the treatment of primary dysmenorrhoea. BJOG 2005; 112: 466–9.

19. Dmowski WP, Gebel H, Braun DP. Decreased apoptosis and sensitivity to macrophage mediated cytolysis of endometrial cells in endometriosis. Hum Reprod Update 1998; 4: 696–701.

20. Meresman GF, Vighi S, Buquet RA et al. Apoptosis and expression of Bcl-2 and Bax in eutopic endometrium from women with endometriosis. Fertil Steril 2000; 74: 760–6.

21. Dmowski WP, Ding J, Shen J et al. Apoptosis in endometrial glandular and stromal cells in women with and without endometriosis. Hum Reprod 2001; 16: 1802–8.

22. Borras M, Leclercq G. Modulatory effect of nonesterified fatty acids on structure and binding characteristics of oestrogen receptor from MCF-7 human breast cancer cells. J Recept Res 1992; 12: 463–84.

23. Gazvani M, Smith L, Haggarty P et al. High omega-3:omega-6 fatty acid ratios in culture medium reduce endometrial-cell survival in combined endometrial gland and stromal cell cultures from women with and without endometriosis. Fertil Steril 2001; 76: 717–22.

24. Haggans CJ, Travellie EJ, Thomas W et al. The effect of flaxseed and wheat bran consumption on urinary oestrogen metabolites in premenopausal women. Epid Bio Prev 2000; 9: 719–25.

25. Gokhale LB. Curative treatment of primary (spasmodic) dysmenorrhoea. Indian J Med Res 1996; 103: 227–31.

26. Fontana-Klatber H, Hogg B. Therapeutic effects of magnesium in dysmenorrhoea. Schweiz Runhdsch Med Prax 1990; 79: 491–4.

27. McLachlan JA, Simpson E, Martin M. Endocrine disrupters and female reproductive health. Best Pract Res Clin Endocrinol Metab 2006; 20: 63–75.

28. Gibbons A. Dioxin tied to endometriosis. Science 1993; 262: 1373.

29. Leone N, Courbon D, Ducimetiere P, Zureik M. Zinc, copper and magnesium and risks for all-cause, cancer, and cardiovascular mortality. Epidemiology 2006; 17: 308–14.

30. Guymer RH, Chong FW. Modifiable risk factors for age-related macular degeneration. Med J Aust 2006; 184: 455–8.

31. Holness MJ, Greenwood GK, Smith ND, Sugden MC. Diabetogenic impact of long-chain omega-3 fatty acids on pancreatic beta-cell function and the regulation of endogenous glucose production. Endocrinology 2003; 144: 3958–68.

Appendix

COMPLEMENTARY AND ALTERNATIVE TREATMENT FOR ENDOMETRIOSIS

There is evidence from two systematic reviews that high-frequency transcutaneous electrical nerve stimulation (TENS), acupuncture, vitamin B_1 and magnesium may help to relieve dysmenorrhoea[1,2]. Whether such treatments are effective in endometriosis-associated dysmenorrhoea is unknown.

Many women with endometriosis report that nutritional and complementary therapies such as reflexology, traditional Chinese medicine, herbal treatments, homeopathy, etc. do improve pain symptoms. Whilst there is no evidence from randomised controlled trials in endometriosis to support these treatments, they should not be ruled out if the woman feels that they could be beneficial to her overall pain management and/or quality of life, or work in conjunction with more traditional therapies.

PROGESTERONE CREAM

There is no evidence that progesterone cream is effective in the treatment of endometriosis. The dose absorbed is minimal, and does not produce amenorrhoea. In clinical trials, the dose was insufficient to result in a withdrawal bleed after a course of oestrogen.

PATIENT SUPPORT GROUPS

Patient self-help groups can provide invaluable counselling, support and advice.

Endometriosis UK
50 Westminster Palace Gardens
Artillery Row
London SW1P 1RR
UK
Tel 0207 222 2781
Freephone helpline 0808 808 2227
enquiries@endometriosis-uk.org
www.endo.org.uk

Endometriosis SHE Trust (UK)
14 Moorland Way
Lincoln LN6 7JW
UK
Tel/fax 0870 774 3665/4
Shetrust@shetrust.org.uk
www.shetrust.org.uk

Endometriosis Association
8585 N. 75th Place
Milwaukee, WI 53223
USA
Tel +1 414 355 2200
Fax +1 414 355 6065
endo@endometriosisassn.org
www.endometriosisassn.org

Endometriosis Research Center
World Headquarters
630 Ibis Drive
Delray Beach, FL 33444
USA
Tel +1 561 274 7442
www.endocenter.org

Human Fertilisation and Embryology Authority
21 Bloomsbury Street
London WC1B 3HF
UK
Tel 0207 291 8200
Fax 0207 291 8201
Licenses and regulates fertility treatment in the United Kingdom. Produces a free infertility and IVF guide.
admin@hfea.gov.uk
www.hfea.gov.uk

Infertility Network UK
Charter House
43 St Leonards Road
Bexhill-on-Sea
East Sussex TN40 1JA
UK
Tel 08701 188088
A national self-help support group for people with infertility.

British Association for Adoption and Fostering
Saffron House
6-10 Kirby Street
London EC1N 8TS
Tel 0207 421 2600
Fax 0207 421 2601
mail@baaf.org.uk
www.baaf.org.uk
The leading UK charity working for children separated from their birth families.

Adoption UK (formerly PPIAS Parent to Parent Information on Adoption Services)
Lower Boddington
Daventry
Northants NN11 6YB
UK
Tel 01327 260195
Fax 01327 263565
An organisation providing help and support for those with any queries concerning adoption.

Relate (central office)
Herbert Gray College
Little Church Street
Rugby CV21 3AP
UK
Tel 01788 573241
www.Relate.org.uk
Offers counselling for those seeking help with relationship difficulties.

REFERENCES

1. Proctor ML, Murphy PA. Herbal and dietary therapies for primary and secondary dysmenorrhoea. Cochrane Database Syst Rev 2001; (2): CD002124.

2. Proctor ML, Smith CA, Farquhar CM, Stones RW. Transcutaneous electrical nerve stimulation and acupuncture for primary dysmenorrhoea. Cochrane Database Syst Rev 2002; (1): CD002123.

Index

adenomyosis
    MRI 85
    ultrasound appearance *28*, 85, *89, 90, 93*
adhesions
    bowel *68, 69, 70*
    and infertility 11, 12
    ovarian 45, *46*
adolescents, endometriosis–associated pain 1
aetiology of endometriosis 2–3
age
    and fertility 11
    and implant characteristics 40
alternative therapies 111
American Fertility Society (AFS) classification system 35
American Society for Reproductive Medicine revised classification *36*
anastrazole 60
angiogenesis 6
animal models 14
anti-endometrial antibodies 6, 13
antioxidants 106
apoptosis 6
appendix, endometriosis of *16, 17*
aromatase inhibitors 60
aromatase P450 messenger RNA expression 26
asoprisnil 60
assisted reproduction 13, 51, 54–6, *54, 55, 56*
atypical implants, histological characteristics 37, *38*
autoantibodies 6

barium enemas 29–30
biopsy 63
blood perfusion studies 88, *95*
buserelin 51, 59
B vitamins 107

CA 125 25–6
Caesarean section scars, endometriotic deposits in *21, 83*
celecoxib 57
cell-mediated immunity 2, 3, 6
Cerazette 59
cervical endometriosis *16*
chocolate cysts *see* endometriomas
classical implants, histological characteristics 37, *38*
classification of endometriosis 35, *36*
clinical features of endometriosis 9–24
    extrapelvic disease *see* extrapelvic endometriosis

infertility *see* infertility associated with endometriosis
    miscarriage rates 15
    natural history 9
    pain *see* pelvic pain associated with endometriosis
    symptoms 1, 9–10, *10*
clinical findings 25–33
    endometriosis sites 25, *26*
    radiological appearances *see* radiology
    serum markers 25–6
coelomic metaplasia theory 2
colonic endometriosis *18, 19*, 26, *79–81*
colour Doppler imaging (CDI) 86–7, *90*
combined oral contraceptive pill (COC) 54, 57–8, *58*
complementary therapies 111
computed tomography (CT) 27, 29
conception
    endometriosis severity and 11
    endometriosis treatment and 12, 14–15
    see also infertility associated with endometriosis
corpus luteal cysts *47*
cyclo-oxygenase (COX)-2 inhibitors 57
cytokines 6

danazol 9, 51, 59
Depo-Provera 58
dermoid cyst *88*
Δ^6-desaturase 105, *106*, 107
diagnosis of endometriosis
    laparoscopic appearance 35–7, *37*, 45, *64, 66*
    see also clinical findings; histology
diaphragmatic endometriosis *22, 23, 82*
diet *see* nutrition in endometriosis management
dioxins 107
docosahexaenoic acid (DHA) *106*, 107
dysmenorrhoea, aetiology 10–11
dyspareunia 10

economic costs of endometriosis 1, 10
eicosanoid imbalance 105
endocrine abnormalities and infertility in endometriosis 12–13
endometrial cells in culture 3, *3*
endometriomas
    diagnosis 25, *26*, 45, *47*
    formation 45
    risk of malignancy score 48, *48*
    surgical treatment 47–8, *47, 49, 71, 72, 74*
    ultrasound appearance 26–7, *27, 28, 29, 86, 87, 89*

epidemiology of endometriosis 1–2, *2*, 10
episiotomy scars, endometriosis in *21, 82, 83*
expectant management of endometriosis 77
extrapelvic endometriosis
   incidence 15
   intestinal tract 15–18, *16–20*, 25, 29–30, *76–81*
   pulmonary and thoracic 21–3, *22, 23*, 75, *82*
   surgical scar-associated 18, 21, *21, 22*, 82–3
   urinary tract 18

fallopian tubes 66
fertility
   influence of age 11
   see also assisted reproduction; infertility associated with
      endometriosis
fibrinolytic system involvement in endometriosis 5–6
fibroblast growth factor 6
flaxseed 105
foods
   nutritional content of 106
   see also nutrition in endometriosis management
functional cysts 45

gamete intrafallopian tube transfer (GIFT) 13, 54
genetics and endometriosis 2, 7
gestrinone 9, 51, 59
β-glucoronidase 107
gonadotrophin releasing hormone agonists 59–60
gonadotrophin releasing hormone antagonists 61
goserelin acetate 59
growth factors 6

haemorrhagic implants
   evolution 40
   histological characteristics 37, *39*
   ovarian 45
healed implants 39
histology
   cyclical changes 5
   evolution of implants 40, *40*
   ovarian endometriosis 40, *40, 41*
   rectovaginal endometriosis 41–2, *42*
   types of implant 5, 37–40, *37, 38, 39*
hormonal control of endometriotic tissue 5
hormone replacement therapy (HRT) after oophorectomy 74
humoral immunity changes in endometriosis 6
hydroureter, ultrasound images *30*

iatrogenic transplantation of endometrial cells 3, *3*
ibuprofen 57
immunological factors
   changes in humoral and cell-mediated immunity 6
   in endometriosis-associated infertility 13
   in susceptibility to endometriosis 2, 3
immunoscintigraphy 30, *31, 32*
incidence of endometriosis 1, 10, 15
infertility associated with endometriosis 11
   adhesions 11, 12
   in animal models 14
   conception rates and disease severity 11
   effects of endometriosis treatment 12, 14–15, 51–2, 54
   possible mechanisms *12*
      abnormal oocytes 13–14

   endocrine abnormalities 12–13
      immune abnormalities 13
      peritoneal fluid factors 13
   see also assisted reproduction
inflammation associated with endometriosis 6
interleukin 1 (IL-1) 6
interleukin 2 (IL-2) 49
intestinal tract endometriosis 15–18, *16–20*, 25, 29–30,
    76–81
intracytoplasmic sperm injection (ICSI) *13*
intrauterine insemination (IUI) 54
in vitro fertilization (IVF) 13, 54, 55–6, *55*

laparoscopic uterosacral nerve ablation (LUNA) 63, 72, *73–4*
laparoscopy
   appearance of endometriosis 35–7, *37*, 45, *64, 66*
   effects on pelvic pain 51, 63, 67, 71, 72, 74
   endometrioma management 48, 71, *72*
   inspection procedure 63, *64, 65, 66*
   presacral neurectomy 72, 74
   treatment modalities 63
   uterine nerve ablation 63, 72, *73–4*
   see also surgical treatment of endometriosis
laparotomy 74
laser ablation 63
levonorgestrel-releasing intrauterine system 59
lifestyle factors 107
luprorelide/leuprorelin acetate 58–9, *59*
luteinised unruptured follicle (LUF) syndrome 12
lymphatic spread of endometriosis 3

macrophages and endometriosis 11
magnesium supplementation 107
magnetic resonance imaging (MRI) 29, *31*, 85
malignant change within endometriosis 77, *84*
medical treatment of endometriosis 51, 57–61
   combined with surgical treatment 54, 75
   effects on fertility 14, 51, 54
   future treatments 60–1
   gestogens and antigestogens 58–9
   gonadotrophin releasing hormone agonists 59–60
   modes of action *58*
   non-steroidal anti-inflammatory drugs 57
   oral contraceptive pill 54, 57–8, *58*
   side-effects *58*
medroxyprogesterone acetate (MPA) 9, 51, 58
mefenamic acid 57
menstruation
   cumulative menstruation and risk of endometriosis 2
   retrograde 2, 3, 10
metaplasia of coelomic epithelium 2
mifepristone 60
miscarriage rates and endometriosis 15

naferelin 59
naproxen 57
natural history of endometriosis 9
nodular implants 39
non-steroidal anti-inflammatory drugs (NSAIDs) 57
nutrition in endometriosis management 105–9
   dietary modifications 105, *106*
   recommendations 108
   supplements 106–7

OC 125 immunoscintigraphy 30, *31, 32*
oestrogen metabolism, effects of dietary flaxseed 105
oestrogen receptors 5
omega 3 fatty acids 105, *106,* 107
omega 6 fatty acids 105, *106*
oocyte abnormalities and endometriosis-associated
 infertility 13–14
oophorectomy 74, *74*
oral contraceptive pill 54, 57–8, *58*
oral Provera 58
ovarian cancer and endometriosis 7
ovarian endometriosis 45–9
 endometriomas
  diagnosis 25, *26,* 45, *47*
  formation 45
  risk of malignancy score 48, *48*
  surgical treatment 47–8, *47, 49,* 71, *72,* 74
  ultrasound appearance 26–7, *27, 28, 29,* 86, *87, 89*
 histopathology 40, *40, 41,* 45
 superficial haemorrhagic implants 45
ovarian stimulation with intrauterine insemination 54
oxidative stress 106

pain *see* pelvic pain associated with endometriosis
papular implants, histological characteristics 37, *38, 39*
pathogenesis of endometriosis 2–3
patient support groups 111–12
pelvic endometriosis
 clinical findings 25, *26*
 defined 15
pelvic pain associated with endometriosis
 aetiology 10–11
 complementary/alternative therapies 111
 correlation with location of deep infiltrating disease 68
 during pregnancy 15
 economic costs 1, 10
 effects of surgery 51, 63, 67, 71, *72,* 74
 medical treatment
  gestogens and antigestogens 58–9
  gonadotrophin releasing hormone agonists 59–60
  non-steroidal anti-inflammatory drugs 57
  oral contraceptive pill 57–8
pelvis, normal view *11*
peritoneal fluid of women with endometriosis 6, 13
phytoestrogens 105
platelet-derived growth factor 6
pouch of Douglas 12, 27, 29, *65*
pregnancy and endometriosis 15, 56, *56*
presacral neurectomy 72
prevalence of endometriosis 1–2, *2,* 10
probiotics 107
progesterone antagonists 60
progesterone cream 111
progesterone receptors in endometriotic tissue 5
progestins 58–9
progestogen-only contraceptive pills 59
programmed cell death 6
prostaglandins in the aetiology of dysmenorrhoea 11
proteolytic capacity of endometriotic tissue 6
proteomics 7
pulmonary endometriosis 21, 23

radiology
 barium enemas 29–30
 computed tomography 27, 29
 immunoscintigraphy 30, *31, 32*
 MRI 29, *31*
 sigmoidoscopy 30
 ultrasound *see* ultrasound assessment of endometriosis
rectovaginal endometriosis
 clinical case 102–3, *102–3*
 clinical findings 25, *26*
 histology and morphology 41, *42*
 response to hormonal treatment 42
red lesions 40
renal endometriosis 18
retrograde menstruation 2, 3, 10
risk factors for endometriosis 2
risk of malignancy index (RMI) scoring system 48, *48*
rofecoxib 57

selective progesterone receptor modulators 60
self-help groups 111–12
serum markers for endometriosis 25–6
sex hormone binding globulin (SHBG) 105
sigmoid colon, endometriosis of *18, 26*
sigmoidoscopy 30
single sweep (Voluson) technology 88, 90
steroid receptors in endometriotic tissue 5
stress 107
superovulation with intrauterine insemination 54
surgery, dissemination of endometrial cells during 3
surgical scar-associated endometriosis 18, 21, *21, 22,* 82–3
surgical treatment of endometriosis 63–84
 combined with medical treatment 54, 75
 effects on fertility 12, 51–2, 54
 effects on pelvic pain 51, 63, 67, 71, *72,* 74
 endometrioma management 47–8, *47, 49,* 71, *72,* 74
 laparotomy 74
 minimal/mild disease 67, *67, 68*
 moderate/severe disease 68, *68, 69–71*
 oophorectomy 74, *74*
 preoperative assessment 67
 recurrent disease 75–6
 see also laparoscopy
symptoms of endometriosis 1, 9–10, *10*

thoracic endometriosis 21, *22, 23,* 75, 82
three-dimensional architecture of endometriosis 39–40, *39*
three-dimensional ultrasound *29, 30,* 87–8, *91, 92–3, 94*
trans fatty acids 105, *106*
treatment of endometriosis
 complementary and alternative 111
 nutrition and lifestyle 105–9
 principles 51–6
 see also medical treatment of endometriosis; surgical treatment
  of endometriosis
triptorelin 59
tumour necrosis factor (THF) 6

ultrasound assessment of endometriosis 85–104
 blood perfusion studies 88, *95*
 clinical cases 90, *93–4, 97–103,* 100, *102, 103*
 colour Doppler imaging 86–7, *90*
 endometriomas 26–7, *27, 28, 29,* 86, *87, 89*

grey-scale (G-S) appearances 85, *86*, *87*, *88*
scanning techniques 85–6, *89*
single sweep technology 88, 90, *96*
three-dimensional imaging *29*, *30*, 87–8, *91*, *92–3*, *94*
umbilicus, endometriosis associated with *21*, 100, *101*, 102
ureteral endometriosis 18
urinary tract endometriosis 18
uterosacral ligament involvement 25, *26*, *38*

vaginal endometriosis *14*, *15*, 21, *82*
valdecoxib 57

vascular endothelial growth factor (VEGF) 6
vascular spread of endometriosis 3
vesical endometriosis 18
vesicular implants 37, *38*
vitamin B 107
vitamin E 106
Voluson (single sweep) technology 88, 90

white lesions 40

xenoestrogens 107